# Strictly Walk Slimmer Walking: The Perfect Outdoor Pursuit for Perpetual Health

I0450500

PAOLA BASSANESE

ISBN-10: 1507746784
ISBN-13: 978-1507746783

Strictly Walk Slimmer features interviews with:

Angelique Panagos of Angelique Panagos Nutrition, featured in ITV's Sugar
Free Farm
Dominique Antiglio of BeSophro
Joanna Hall, TV fitness expert and Founder of Walkactive
Tracey Cox, Author and TV expert
John Resten of Forage London

# ACKNOWLEDGEMENTS

I am extremely grateful to these wonderful people who contributed to my Indiegogo campaign to get this project off the ground:
Cynthia Given
Ian Tilsed
Charlie Casley
Lorella Terzi

A special thank you to the experts I interviewed for this book:
John Rensten
Angelique Panagos
Dominique Antiglio
Tracey Cox
Joanna Hall

## FOREWORD

Strictly Walk Slimmer is an informal guide to the benefits of walking, featuring interviews with thought leaders in the health and wellness fields, plus a list of healthy eating recipes created by the author in her (very tiny!) kitchen over the years.

## DISCLAIMER

The information contained in this book should not be considered as medical advice. Lifestyle suggestions in this book are not meant to be a substitute medical advice: always consult a doctor before undertaking any lifestyle changes.

## COPYRIGHT

# CONTENTS

## Table of Contents

## INTRODUCTION

Strictly Walk Slimmer is divided into four sections:

- principles of walking
- discussion about diets
- health benefits of walking and walking activities
- recipes

At the end of the chapters you will find a resources section listing books and useful websites.

# 1 Looking After Your Health

Some people keep fit by lifting weights at the gym; others by running or taking dance classes. I walk. From climbing Machu Picchu in Peru to walking the Gold Trail in Brazil, I have clocked up some serious mileage in my lifetime.

Have you watched the film Wild (Jean-Marc Vallée, 2014) starring Reese Witherspoon? In this film the protagonist, Cheryl Strayed, walks for 1,100 miles on the Pacific Crest Trail to find herself, make sense of her life and take time to grieve the loss of her mother and the collapse of her wedding.

I completed the Inca Trail in Peru in 2004. It was possibly the longest 26 miles I've ever walked, as you are gasping for breath because of the altitude. The highest point is accurately named Dead Woman's Pass at an altitude of 4200 meters or 13776 feet.
You certainly don't need to go to those extremes to embrace walking as exercise, but consistency is key to make walking your fitness regime of choice.

I walk every day with an average of 50 km a week. Why do I walk? Because I'd rather be out in the fresh air – and I'm not buying into any fad fitness craze or fad diet. As an added bonus, exercising in the fresh air has a rejuvenating effect – it keeps both your skin and your brain younger, and even allows you to meditate and relax.

Is it just me who feels fat and uncomfortable when I see "fitness inspiration" (fitspo) pictures on social media? Is it just me who thinks of all the reasons why I shouldn't aim to have 10% body fat?

Is it just me who thinks there's more to life than counting calories and biceps curls repetitions?

These "fitspo" pictures cluttering our screens are supposed to encourage us to embrace a healthier lifestyle, but in my case they just make me feel like an overweight middle aged woman who has never had a six pack (and has no desire to have one in the future as an old age pensioner). What is your opinion on fad diets, fitness trends and media pressures to be slimmer?

My main goal is to ensure I lead a relatively long and healthy life, and to achieve that I want to manage my cholesterol and blood sugar levels. I want to share with you what I've learned so far and offer you suggestions on what is achievable. I believe that walking is a complete form of exercise that has plenty of health benefits for both mind and body. To ensure my book has a more holistic perspective, I have interviewed a number of experts and researchers on health, nutrition, foraging, meditation and the health benefits of walking, plus I have accessed a large number of publications.

If you, like me, enjoy walking and want to make the most of your available spare time, you will find plenty of information on how walking can have beneficial effects on your overall health and, additionally, there's a number of suggested activities that you can combine with walking to keep your brain engaged too. From foraging to meditation, you will discover new ways of approaching walking that will add more interest to your outdoor pursuits.

Studies found that abdominal fat is linked to degenerative diseases like diabetes and heart failure. Abdominal body fat is more dangerous than overall body fat as measured in the body mass index (BMI): according to a Harvard study, abdominal body fat is the worst type of body fat and it is linked to high cholesterol, stiffness in the arteries (arteriosclerosis), dementia, diabetes and even lung disease.

Although a six pack may be nice to look at and amazing to show proudly in your holiday pictures, what is really important for long-term health is achieving low levels of fat around your internal organs. Lowering the levels of abdominal fat can be achieved by a healthy eating regime and regular exercise, which in this case is walking.

Visceral fat surrounds our organs and can be linked to an excessive response to stress which, in turn, triggers an accumulation of fat, a rise in blood pressure and blood sugar levels, high cholesterol and irregular heart beat.

The most accurate way to measure visceral fat is to do an MRI scan, however a good starting point to understand if you might be at risk is to take your hip-to-waist ratio measurement.

First, measure your waist and your hips in inches; then, divide your waist measurement in inches by your hips measurement in inches. For men, a ratio above 0.95 can indicate a risk of a heart attack or stroke; for women, it is a ratio of 0.85 and above.

There's even a simpler way to measure risk.

If you, like me, are not mathematically inclined, experts say that simply measuring your waist is enough to estimate whether you may have excess abdominal fat and whether you should investigate your risk further.

Following is a table, taken from the Harvard study mentioned above, which gives you an indication of what to look for.

| Waist measurement and risk | Men | Women |
| --- | --- | --- |
| Low risk | 37 inches and below (94 cm and below) | 31.5 inches and below (80 cm and below) |
| Intermediate risk | 37.1–39.9 inches (up to 101 cm) | 31.6–34.9 inches (up to 89 cm) |
| High risk | 40 inches and above (more than 101 cm) | 35 inches and above (more than 89 cm) |

A way to mitigate the risk of developing degenerative diseases if your waist measurement is too high is to lose weight through the correct nutritional intervention from a medical professional and regular exercise.

It is quite normal for weight to fluctuate, so the scales may not always give an accurate picture, whereas measuring your waist gives a fairly accurate reference for risk of diabetes and cardiovascular degenerative diseases.

## I Walk, therefore I Am

Please indulge me while I discuss briefly the genesis of walking as a useful activity to achieve a long and healthy life as well as a way to induce clearer thinking and support learning.

Remember Peripatetic philosophy? Ancient Greek philosophy was borne out of conversations between philosophers and their students, dissecting the nature of reality over extended dialogues and walks. In his book on teaching, Robert Gardner argues that the Greeks made outdoor passing of knowledge to students the gold standard of teaching. In contrast to the soporific nature of teaching in the classroom, Greek philosophers took their students out of the classroom on long walks during which gazing into the horizon was encouraged.

"Insofar as Socrates was a conformist", Gardner argues, "his peripatetic teaching advanced the first steps from indoor lecturing toward outdoor walking and talking. He simply exploited the existing circumstance that the Greeks were suckers for anything that promised to develop a sound mind in a sound body".

Later on in the book we will explore the health benefits of walking for mind and mood. For the time being, it is good to remind ourselves that walking can do wonders for our mental well-being.

## A Perfectly Portable Outdoor Pursuit for Perpetual Health

If walking is a complete form of exercise, then the next step is to ensure we walk every day to gain the maximum benefits from it.

What are your key health goals? Would you like to improve your lung capacity (for example, being able to walk up the stairs without huffing and puffing), to lose weight (but without fad diets), to lower your cholesterol and blood sugar levels?

To get realistic and sustainable results it is essential to plan ahead.

How much spare time can you carve out of your morning, day or evening? If you are to embrace walking as your main form of exercise, daily walks are compulsory (there's no "off day" with walking). The key is not to think of daily walks as a chore but simply as an activity to fit into your day, and it doesn't even require any special equipment.

While not everybody will agree that walking is enough to improve your fitness levels and lose weight, there is a number of research studies that confirm that daily walking help people gain significant health benefits including weight and inch loss. In particular, movement specialist Joanna Hall conducted a scientific study with the South Bank University Sports Performance Laboratory which proved that people using her walking technique achieved significant inch and weight loss. You can learn more about this in Chapter 3.

Studies are showing that there's more to walking than meets the eye: for example, a report from the University of East Anglia (UEA) showed that workers who commute to work either by bike or on foot are more resilient to stress than those who use a car or public transport.

This study compared the habits of 18,000 UK workers who commute daily over a period of 18 years. The majority of the group (73%) commuted by car and 13% walked to work.

The walkers showed lower levels of stress and better health than their more sedentary counterparts.

It's time to look at walking as a way to lose weight but also to keep stress at bay.

## My Experience

I have been measuring daily distances I walked, calories per day and waist/hips size. For the purpose of this book, I kept a food diary for five months of all the foods I ate and all the walking I did each day.

Keeping a food diary can be very educational if done correctly: knowing about calorie intake can be eye-opening when we realise that the foods we considered as being "healthy" may be too calorific to be consumed with abandon.

For example, popcorn is often recommended as a low-calorie snack but what about the popcorn you have at the cinema? Portions can be huge and before you know it you've scoffed 500 calories worth of food that will not keep you full.

Portion control may be something we all need to work on, especially if we consider ready-made dishes which may serve two people but we individually consume all in one meal.

I thought I had a reasonably good diet and I thought I knew how many calories there were approximately in each meal I ate, but it was only when I started tracking my calories that I realised that some days I was exceeding the recommended calorie intake. More importantly, I learned to think twice before having something like a doughnut or a packet of crisps – not just because of its calorie content, but most importantly because this type of food has hardly any nutritional value (more on "empty calories" later). If one jam doughnut has more calories than two scrambled eggs and it will make you feel hungry half an hour after eating it, then it will have to go.

I used the apps MyFitnessPal to keep track of my calories and MapMyWalk to calculate the distances I walked. Of course, there's several fitness apps you can experiment with so choose whichever suits your lifestyle.

A food diary can also be useful to remind ourselves of those snacks we forget to consider as "food" in our day – we conveniently don't remember that packet of crisps we had on the train on our way home from work or those squares of chocolate we had mid-morning as we needed an energy boost. A food diary is a tool to observe our eating behaviours and to evaluate whether we need to improve in some areas like having more fruit and vegetables, or even more water. You can also use a food diary app to compare ready meals with home made meals: it can even incentivise you to find creative ways to make a recipe healthier.

To give you an example: you can swap a take-away or frozen pizza (between 600 and 1000 calories) to a home made pizza using a tortilla wrap as a base, with a tomato, ham and mozzarella topping (300 calories).

As long as keeping a food diary does not become an obsession, being aware of your food intake can make a big difference to your weight.

Keeping track of your walking can be a great motivational tool: I personally prefer using an integrated map app like Map My Walk to see the connection between kilometers walked and calories burned. Of course, not all calories were created equal (more on that later), but the thought of theoretically being able to, say, burn the calorie equivalent of a Magnum ice cream (or any other food with the same calorie content) by walking at a fast pace for one hour is very appealing.

Over the course of five months, I walked 1057 km and burned 66,600 calories, with a peak of 234 km walked in one month. That is quite a few miles (and a good bunch of calories), right? During my best month I walked 230.5 km: the weather was excellent and I was finding any excuses I could to go out in the fresh air.

On average I walked 200 km a month, i.e., approximately 50 km a week. This works out at about 30 minutes to one hour walking a day. I tend to prefer walking for one continuously but you can break down your daily exercise into 15 minutes chunks, as long as there's some good intensity in your walking technique. To give an example: when I walk for two hours at a medium pace I burned 600 calories (you can burn approximately the same during one hour of Zumba). I know that two hours is a huge investment of your time, but if you were to break it down into 15 minutes chunks you could be clocking that throughout the day.

Because you will be walking every day you may want to keep things interesting by planning a number of different routes or, if you don't have enough time to explore new areas, you can always turn a different corner along your normal route, you never know where it will take you.

During those five months, when I monitored distances and calories on a daily basis, I lost 5kg, which isn't much as what fad diets would promise, as you could be losing that in one month. However, I didn't want to follow a restrictive diet because the risk of gaining the weight back on is very high. The combination of walking and not overeating is a sustainable way to prevent weight gain in the future. What I found very useful about tracking calories (which I then stopped doing as I wanted to depend less on my mobile!) was that it made me very creative in the kitchen, as I experimented with different recipes. You can find a selection of healthy recipes in chapter 4.

You may become best friends with Google Maps (or any other map) while you plan your daily routes. You will also end up exploring your local area more and discover places you didn't know were there before.

## Burning Calories is like Carbon Emission Offsetting: Not a Zero-Sum Game

You may be tempted to think "if I go to a spin class I can eat what I want all day" or "I've had a slice of cake so now I'll need to run for one hour to burn it off".

While it's quite educational to look at calories in meals and have an idea of how much effort it takes to exercise the calorie equivalent of these meals, the body has a completely different type of intelligence that does not compute calories in and calories out the way our mind does.

More importantly, you can't assume that weight loss can be put on a spreadsheet and it will show as a linear progression towards your target weight.

Medical studies have revealed that "burning fat" is a theoretical concept: when we lose weight, we lose water, fat and lean mass at the same time.

There is a useful tool called Calories per Hour which states that you need to burn 7,716 calories to lose 1 kg of fat. That's quite a challenge to exercise your way to 7,716 calories. Bodies are programmed to hold on to body fat to keep us alive and keep all our internal organs functioning.

Losing weight quickly is like emptying the contents of a heavy backpack you have been carrying. You donate clothes and accessories that used to be in the backpack to charity shops and your rucksack feels lighter. Then, after a while, you start seeing things that you like and you start buying clothes, shoes, souvenirs, presents for friends and the list goes on. You put your purchases in your rucksack and, all of a sudden, and without you realising it, your rucksack is heavy and probably fuller than you started with before giving away its contents initially.

Losing weight slowly but steadily is like wearing a heavy rucksack full of stones (I am borrowing this image from counselling theories). Every so often, you take one stone out of your rucksack and you walk on.

Then you do that again with another stone, but you don't rush to empty your rucksack all at once: you adjust to the new weight and carry on. Your rucksack feels lighter. You still need a few stones in your rucksack for resistance so you don't sway from side to side:

that is your normal weight.

Which of these game strategies would you choose?

Depending on your age and gender, hormones play an important role in weight gain.

Women going through the menopause may experience unexplained weight gain, particularly around their waist.

The right nutrition, managing stress levels, exercise and good quality sleep can have a beneficial effect on hormones, fat storage in the body and weight. In other words, lifestyle choices influence your health.

Oestrogen, and its component part oestradiol, regulates how fat is stored and is an important hormone for preventing degenerative diseases. Oestradiol contributes to regulate sleeping patterns.

Testosterone levels tend to rise after the menopause and a side effect that needs monitoring is the influence testosterone has on abdominal fat.

**Tips:**
- Aim to walk at least 20 minutes a day
- go for a brisk walk first thing in the morning, if possible. 10-15 minutes is fine but make sure you add more walking throughout the day
- use fitness apps to track your progress
- plan your walking route and make it interesting by finding alternative routes.

# 2 Diet Myths Debunked

I have a theory. According to my theory, guilt could be making people fat. In other words: you are doing great, dieting and exercising, but the guilt from having just one piece of cake shatters your confidence. You lose all hope and you start thinking "I am a failure". You then start to eat your way out of your guilt trip, only to realise that you have started over-eating.

Self-sabotage is the enemy of dieters. Whether it's down to guilt or any other emotion, we need to check what attitude we have towards food.

Both lack of knowledge and too much knowledge of nutrition principles can be detrimental. Ironically, we are bombarded with information about the latest diets and weight loss programmes, but the obesity crisis is still very real. There is also the issue is that some of the free information on nutrition may be sponsored by large food manufacturers or may not be backed by scientific research.

Restrictive diets are, by their nature, only supposed to last for a short period of time (and absolutely under the guidance of a medical professional) and have been designed to address specific health conditions (for example, high cholesterol). The body will fight any long term diet restricting the calorie intake and will hold on to its fat reserves entering a survival mode.

## Why Diets Don't Work

If you search for "why diets don't work" you will find plenty of reasons; as Forbes Magazine succinctly said in an article: "Don't go on a diet".
When it comes to healthy eating, Deepak Chopra in What are you Hungry for says, "The solution is to transform your awareness."
Fad diets are less likely to succeed in keeping the weight down after an initial weight loss. The US Attorney General published a report in an attempt to warn consumers about outlandish weight loss claims from diet companies. After going on a fact-finding mission, the Attorney General report quotes from research into weight loss saying that only 5% of people who had been on a diet managed to keep the weight off in the long term. In fact, most people tend to gain back all the weight they had lost when eating normally (i.e., when they are not following a restrictive diet).
The report also mentions that experts advise you to keep your expectations realistic: losing a pound/ 0.5 kilo a week is safe and sustainable. It also quotes that to achieve this you will need to cut 500 calories a day (3,500 a week) to shed approximately one pound/ half a kilo of fat.
However, we must remember that when we lose weight our body will shed not only fat but also water and lean (muscle) mass. Targeted weight loss is unfortunately not realistic: we can't pick and choose only one area of our body that we want to be leaner.
Diets have been designed to target a specific health condition (diabetes, high cholesterol, epilepsy etc.). They are prescribed by a doctor or other health professional and must be monitored throughout. DYI diets can be dangerous and could lead to long term health problems.
Additionally, social media messages can be confusing. What is a "cheat day"? What is "eating clean"? There's no standard answer to these questions. If a "cheat day" is a day when you are allowed to eat slightly more than your calorie-controlled, food group restricted diet, if you ask different health professionals or fitness experts they will come up with different answers. For some a "cheat day" is to have grilled chicken with steamed carrots and broccoli. Yay! What a feast! It beats having all the "treats" at

Christmas and all Easter chocolate eggs at once! If we look at the terminology, "cheat" is a strong word which evokes emotions of betrayal. "Naughty foods" are also very emotionally charged and associated to feelings of "breaking the rules" so how do these words make us feel when we are breaking our diet to indulge in naughty foods?

There's more: when I hear people (mostly women) saying "I can eat what I want and still be slim", what I think these people really mean is that they forced themselves to like kale chips...

I spoke with nutritionist and nutritional therapist Angelique Panagos to find out more about fad diets and how we can achieve a more balanced approach to healthy eating.

"The problem with diets", she said, "is that we definitely don't seem to be able to sustain them in the long term." This is especially true for the promise of weight loss that comes along with the diet and the fact that the promised shedding of weight will magically happen in a very short time. The strain that crash dieting puts on the body is a serious issue.

"First of all, we are going on a diet and in three months we will have lost the weight, and then what?" Angelique remarked, as a reminder to all of us that to achieve balance we need a maintenance plan to keep the weight off while maintaining a healthy lifestyle in the long term.

Is the rapid slimming promised by a fad diet a natural way for the body to lose weight? The answer is: obviously not. However, we do need some form of diet or healthy eating regime to counteract the current obesity crisis in most of the Western world. "If we don't do something about weight loss we are headed for disaster. We could all do with some sort of weight loss plan if we are slightly overweight and if we haven't been careful about what we eat" Angelique said, and recommended to stay away from fad diets and to do your research into nutrition and how to get the best nutrients and nourishment from food.

"There isn't enough evidence or enough research to support these fad diets", Angelique remarks, and explains that we are all individual with very specific nutritional needs. A one-size-fits-all approach won't work but what can we do if we can't go and see a nutritionist to get a personalised diet plan?

If we make the assumption that the general population is quite unhealthy on average and those who are unhealthy have varying degrees of disease (from obesity to diabetes), how can we say that the same diet will work for everybody across the board? It won't, because you need to sit down with each individual person and find out what type of eating plan will work for them.

Angelique is used to seeing clients who come to her saying they have tried "every single diet there is" and weren't successful in keeping the weight down in the long term. That says a lot about the shortcomings of popular diets, especially those that are endorsed by celebrities.

Because not everybody can afford to see a nutritionist, here are some guidelines that we can all follow to be better informed about diet and nutrition.

**Diets under the Microscope**

Angelique recommends starting to get information on healthy eating from good quality blogs backed by scientific research.
Her personal favourites are:

- I Quit Sugar
- Against All Grain

These blogs are quite specific and look at healing the body from autoimmune conditions, however you can take inspiration from the recipes and practical advice (including how to make healthy packed lunches and snacks).

Best selling diet books focus on a specific angle to achieve weight loss (mostly with a short term vision): from portion control to excluding food groups, to cutting fat.

Among the best sellers, a selection of diet books are:

- Atkins diet
- Paleo diet
- GI diet
- Blood Type diet
- 5:2 diet
- Vegan diet
- Zone diet

If you look at customer comments in online reviews of all diet books, the results tend to sum up as this: fast weight loss in week one, slower weight loss in week two, weight fluctuations in weeks three and four. Maintenance programmes may or may not be included in diet books but even if they are, how many people will read that chapter on the maintenance plan and stick to it? There's the issue of having to change ingrained behaviours and long term habits that can be hard to break.

Genuine comments (i.e. not sponsored reviews) from reviewers of best-selling diet books tend to point out that you can't diet for the rest of your life because you will end up relapsing and therefore going back to your old, less healthy habits (the path of least resistance).

Reviewers also mentioned the undesired side-effects of some fad diets: these side-effects can range from stomach upsets to bad breath, from constipation to diarrhoea, moods swings and headaches, even insomnia and irritability.

Of all the diets and their permutations, probably the 5:2 approach seems to attract the least amount of criticism from the media and the general public. Popularised by a BBC Horizon programme presented by Dr Michael Mosley, the intermittent fasting diet or 5:2 diet became extremely popular very quickly in the UK and people started reporting positive results. When I asked Angelique what she thought about the 5:2 diet, she said that the restricting of calories has the effect of lessening the insulin response and therefore balancing our blood sugar. The by-product is weight reduction and, therefore, better health in the longer term, as long as you make permanent lifestyle changes. However, because this diet emerged only in recent years, there is not enough scientific research to demonstrate its effectiveness across the board.

**Diets at a Glance**

According to the New England Journal of Medicine, portion control and limiting the intake of calories is essential for weight loss, regardless of which food groups are included or excluded.

In the study, 811 overweight adults were given a diet selected at random. The diets had different proportions of carbohydrates, fat and protein. The proportions of energy from fat, protein, and carbohydrates in the four diets were as follows:

- diet 1 had 20% carbohydrates, 15% fat, and 65% protein;
- diet 2 had 20% carbohydrates, 25% fat, and 55% protein;
- diet 3 had 40% carbohydrates, 15% fat, and 45% protein;
- diet 4 had 40% carbohydrates, 25% fat, and 35% protein.

The diets had similar ingredients and were designed to support cardiovascular health. Participants had to adhere to their diets for two years.

The aim of the study was to calculate weight loss in participants according to which diet worked best. The interim results after six months demonstrated that all participants, regardless of which diet they followed, had lost 6 kg on average (about 7% weight loss from their starting weight) and then they started gaining some weight back after 12 months.

After two years, all participants, regardless of which diet they were following, had lost a total of approximately 3 kg. Not all participants completed the trial (80% did), and those who followed the diet for the full two years lost on average of 4 kg. Similarities were also found when participants were asked about how hungry or how full they felt during their diet.

The overall results showed an improvement in the reduction of health risks associated to body fat and blood sugar levels. The study also showed that weight loss will plateau at some point.

Why are we relying on fad diets to give us a temporary "high" fooling us into thinking that we have solved all our weight and health problems after, say, following a restrictive and punishing diet for three months? Why can't we just stick to a long term healthy eating plan instead?

Eating regimes like the paleo diet have attracted criticism because of their restrictive nature, so how can we make better food decisions?

Angelique explained that "people get confused when they hear 'paleo diet', 'hunter-gatherer diet': they feel they need to be eating a lot of meat and that comes from the Atkins diet" (which relies on meat and fat while being low on fruit and vegetables). "Paleo is not that. Paleo is eating a balanced diet with lots of vegetables and proteins and you get different of types of paleo: some include grains, while others are very strict and don't." She recommends avoiding processed, man-made grains when possible as they are not rich in nutrients: "they are more anti-nutrients than anything else." From white bread and pasta to sugary breakfast cereals, man-made grains will cause a sudden spike of sugar in the blood, causing lack of energy and food cravings shortly afterwards.

Angelique explained her own philosophy about food and eating: "I'm not into 'strict-anything'. I don't do it myself so I can't tell anyone to do it". What she does as a practitioner is to take the best from the healthy eating plans available and create a personalised plan for her clients.

## Much ado about 5:2?

The basis of the 5:2 diet, Angelique explained, is the restricting of calories, which is in effect a lessening the insulin response. Therefore the 5:2 diet aims to balance our blood sugar levels while reducing weight and making ourselves healthier in the process. Every time we eat there is an element of "endotoxicity" (release of toxins), which is a natural by-product of breaking down food in the digestive system.

We have become so used to eating constantly, without even realising we do that. Food has never been so abundant and you can grab anything you fancy eating easily from any shop. The premise of the 5:2 diet is to reduce the food intake to 500 calories a day a couple of times a week and this can have both positive and negative effects. However, more research is needed: is the 5:2 diet an eating regime for life? When do you stop dieting and go back to "normal"? What are the contraindications?

5:2 is the "new kid on the block" of diets and because no one has been doing it for 10 years we don't have enough data about what exactly happens in the body. Angelique added: "my own father did the 5:2 and he did drop the weight, and his weight has stabilised now because I put him on a maintenance way of eating". The maintenance plan includes only one day of calorie restriction and on that day you would normally have your breakfast later than usual, then one main meal combining lunch and dinner together –

therefore making it a 6:1 plan. Of course, never start a DYI diet without first talking to a medical professional to get professional advice.

Insulin is a major driver in weight gain and ill health. "My concern with the 5:2" Angelique said "is in doing it incorrectly." The BBC programme that first popularised the 5:2 diet showed that you put it all the allocated 500 calories of a typical "fast day" in one meal. Angelique believes you can improve on that by splitting those calories into two meals choosing good quality foods, namely dark green vegetables, protein and some fat.

Angelique suggested: "you could maybe start your day with a green smoothie, high in calcium, high in iron, throw in some flaxseed, some coconut oil for the fat and protein, then having a small lunch like having an egg with some vegetables and then for dinner having some fish and vegetables." She also suggested keeping 5 hours in between meals and not going more than that without food. "When we have more than 5 hours in between meals we go into low blood sugar (hypoglycaemia), so that's when we stimulate the adrenaline and cortisol from the adrenal glands to raise our blood sugar."

So how can we start eating more healthily and how can we stick to it? Angelique's reply was that it all depends on the individual: if you feel jittery if you don't eat after 3 hours from your last meal, then your food prescription is to eat every 3-4 hours. But if you can go 4 hours without eating then your food prescription is 4-5 hours. In any case, the recommendation is not to go longer than that 5 hour mark. Angelique sums this up as follows: "if we are talking about optimal health we are also talking about that we can't do everything perfectly every day." The 80/20 rule applies: as long as we are in control at least 80% of the time doing really well with our food intake, then the remaining 20% of the time will not be a problem as our body can be quite forgiving.

The next question that springs to mind after talking about gaps between meals is how do we recognise a natural hunger signal and how do we know that we are eating something because we are bored instead of being truly hungry.

Angelique reminds us to take a step back and prioritise: the first thing we need to do is to get out of an existing stress response. When we are stressed we are more likely to overeat or misinterpret our hunger signals. In this situation, breathing techniques and dynamic relaxation like Sophrology can be very effective to lower our stress levels. We will talk about Sophrology later on. Relaxation techniques allow you to connect again with your body and listen to its needs.

The first thing you need to do when a hunger pang strikes is to have a bit of water, aiming for at least a whole cup of water. Then you need to ask yourself how much water do you drink in a day: you may be surprised at how little water you are drinking.

On the other hand, if you are really thirsty all the time it is a good idea to check for blood sugar and diabetes risk.

Another useful check you can do to assess whether you are hungry or not would be to notice if you are salivating: when we are hungry our body naturally starts our first digestive process, which is to produce saliva. This process gets our digestive juices going and we are ready to eat food.

We only need to look at nature to remind ourselves of this basic principle: when animals are hungry they start salivating.

Thirdly, if you are starting to feel jittery or light-headed, then that's not boredom. Angelique said: "I think it's really taking note of those signals". She expressed concerns about what I would call 'machismo in the office' because we never stop, not even for basic functions like going to the loo and taking breaks. "Going to the loo takes time out of our day!" joked Angelique; "we stop the basics of survival, that's when we start getting these signals crossed. Keeping to eating every 5 hours (unless you're hypoglycaemic), then you start realising that you don't need those snacks in between meals". She recommended, if you really need to eat between meal as you are feeling faint, to snack on something healthy like nuts and seeds, some fruit, some hummus and vegetable sticks. "Because I've been there myself" Angelique added, "I can totally relate. At times I would be sitting at my desk, raring to go to the bathroom, but I carried on typing!"

According to Angelique being productive and getting things done requires organisation and a good level of awareness: if you're thinking about a normal function like going to the toilet you will end up feeling distracted so take care of the basics first.

Being prepared also means planning some time to get up from your desk for a few minutes – that little bit of movement is going to be really good for your back and legs while giving your eyes some rest as you will not be staring at the screen continuously. You're doing yourself a favour by simply getting up and moving around.

Many people say that they don't have time to go out and eat something, whether it's at lunchtime or simply grabbing a snack. At least we have drawers in our office desks so we can keep healthy foods there. "All you need to do is stock up once a month or once a week on the right types of food to have at hand" said Angelique. She assured that this doesn't mean that you should never have chocolate again. Of course there are different types of chocolate so when you need your fix choose organic dark chocolate instead of heavily processed chocolate with hydrogenated fat.

Angelique's best tip is to drink more water: "I really recommend to people to fill a bottle, preferably a glass bottle, not a plastic one, and keep it on your desk to see how much you are drinking. We need to be having 35ml per kilo of body weight per day. You can work out your own water prescription what you need to be drinking and that can include herbal teas but that definitely does not include caffeine."

Ask yourself when and why you need to have coffee: if you wake up and the first thing you do is have a cup of coffee with, say, 3 sugars and some milk you are having the calorie equivalent a liquid meal. Unfortunately not only you won't feel satisfied and will still feel hungry after having a coffee but you will also going to raise your blood sugar levels. Angelique explained: "I advise people to first have breakfast and 10 minutes later to have one cup of coffee. If you can't function without coffee then we really need to look at what's going on and why you are not able to function without coffee and how we can get a deeper sleep so that you are more refreshed. Are you not functioning because you are not rested?"

Listening to what our bodies need also means that we have to check whether we are on a roller-coaster ride of sugar highs and lows. We may not even remember what "normal" feels like and have become addicted to running on nervous energy. Angelique explained: "there's also an element of people not wanting to let go of the habit. We are creatures of habit."

A former 8-coffees-a-day person herself, now caffeine-free

Angelique acknowledged that not everybody can give up coffee that easily (or at all, like me!) and she admitted that there's nothing wrong with one cup of good quality coffee a day followed by some water.

Continuing on the theme of sugar and how it affects the body, we need to talk about alcohol: "we live in a very social world" remarked Angelique: "we have an excuse for every season: in summer – we should sit outside and have a drink,... we have to drink for Christmas" and so on. Angelique stated that alcohol is an anti-nutrient, which causes a spike in your blood sugar levels and triggering an insulin response, plus it's high in calories.

It's not just the alcohol that we consume: Angelique expressed her concern that we are adding Red Bull, Coca-Cola, diet drinks full of aspartame, cordials to alcohol which multiplies the sugar and toxicity make up of a drink. Angelique suggested "having 5 alcohol-free nights a week, 6 if possible, and on the nights we are drinking to alternate drinks with a glass of water, drink water socially (put it in a wine glass if you have to) as if it was your drink and slow down that process of over-indulging." Sip water between sips of wine or other alcohol during a night out, celebration or even during a meal at home.

"People need to stop counting calories and start counting toxins" remarked Angelique. Sure, there are more calories in an apple than there is in a so called "healthy" cereal bar which is likely to be full of sugar. Weight for weight there might be less calories in the cereal bar but the effect those calories have on the body is completely different. An apple is 90 calories and a healthy breakfast bars is 56 calories – which one to choose? The apple, which has healing properties, or the sugar-laden cereal bar? Be wary of heavily advertised food products: "I don't see the humble apple having its own advert with any celebrities endorsing it!" said Angelique.

**Weight loss diets: pros and cons**

Let's look at the most popular weight loss diets out there and their pros and cons.

| Diet | Useful for | Risks | Source |
|---|---|---|---|
| **Atkins** | Short term weight loss and control of diabetes. | Contraindicated for those affected by kidney disease. Risk of developing eating disorders due to carbohydrates cravings. | *Dr Atkins New Diet Revolution: The No-hunger, Luxurious Weight Loss Plan That Really Works!* by Robert C Atkins |
| **Paleo** | Weight loss and reliance on eating natural foods, i.e., avoiding processed foods. | Over-reliance on red meat and cutting out whole grains completely are associated to risk of developing heart disease and some cancers. Risk of developing eating disorders due to carbohydrates cravings. | *The Paleo Diet: Lose Weight and Get Healthy by Eating the Foods You Were Designed to Eat* by Loren Cordain |
| **GI Diet** | The key benefit is a reduction in blood sugar level fluctuations and therefore insulin levels. It reduces the risk of developing heart conditions and diabetes. | Risk of hypoglycaemia. Some low GI foods are unhealthy. | *The Gi Diet: The Glycemic Index; The Easy, Healthy Way to Permanent Weight Loss* by Rick Gallop |

| Diet | Useful for | Risks | Source |
|---|---|---|---|
| Blood type diet | Weight loss. According to the blood type diet theory, our ancestors chose some foods instead of others depending on whether the whole tribe was nomadic or not. | Not enough research available. Restricting whole food groups can lead to nutritional deficiencies. | *Eat Right 4 Your Type* by Peter D'Adamo |
| 5:2 diet | Intermittent fasting can lower cholesterol, blood sugar levels and blood pressure. Also credited for increasing life span and protecting against Alzheimer's. | Can affect sleep patterns and cause irritability. Contraindicated in cases of eating disorders. Not enough research available. | *The Fast Diet: The Secret of Intermittent Fasting – Lose Weight, Stay Healthy, Live Longer* by Dr Michael Mosley |
| Vegan | Weight loss, lower cholesterol levels, lower risk of heart disease and reliance on eating natural foods, when done correctly. | Over-reliance on refined vegan foods (white flour, white rice and pasta etc.) can lead to nutritional deficiencies (iron, vitamin B12 and Omega 3 deficiency). | *Vegan for Life: Everything You Need to Know to Be Healthy and Fit on a Plant-Based Diet* by Jack Norris |
| Zone Diet | In this diet 40% of daily calories should be carbohydrates, 30% protein, 30% fat. It is based on portion control and has some fresh fruit and vegetables. The diet was designed for people allergic to yeasts and grains. | Rapid weight gain when stopping the diet. The diet limits some sources of essential nutrients. | *Enter The Zone – A Dietary Road Map to Lose Weight Permanently* by Barry Sears |

## Not all Calories were Created Equal

The myth of a low-calorie diet as the best way to lose weight is just that: a myth. In other words: beware of fad diets, "low-fat" foods, "low-calorie" foods and just any trend that grabs the headlines.

Gram for gram, calories from sugar have a completely different impact on the body than calories from vegetables and protein.

We are familiar with the concept of "empty calories": from sugary drinks to processed foods, this type of calories doesn't give the necessary nourishment to sustain the body but it can contribute to weight and fat gain.

Knowing more about the right type of calories we should be getting, avoiding "empty calories" and limiting our sugar intake are the foundations of a good diet for long term health. The National Diabetes Information Clearinghouse (NDIC), a service of the National Institute of Diabetes and Digestive and Kidney Diseases (NIDDK) and National Institutes of Health (NIH) reports that many people may have insulin resistance but may not know about it and may be living with the condition for a number of years, untreated.

Insulin resistance is associated with chronic illness but if you have insulin resistance you can learn to make lifestyle changes to prevent the onset of type 2 diabetes.

We should all be more aware of our lifestyle habits to prevent chronic diseases. A fairly common behaviour is to save your calories from food if you know that you are going to have one or more alcoholic drinks in the evening. In theory it sounds like a good idea, because on paper you are not exceeding the total daily recommended calorie intake. However, as Angelique is reminding us, "you are having empty calories": this means that you are ingesting an anti-nutrient which comes with its own toxic load on the body. The other problem with alcohol is knowing when to stop: most of the time it's too late when we realise we have had too much to drink.

"That's the whole thing about body awareness: if you are really serious about weight loss and maintaining your weight then you are going to make the right change – the change I would like to see people make is not change for this month, but change for life" is

Angelique's message. Again, it's not all doom and gloom: "once you get into this habit – and we are creatures of habit – then you'll see that you can go out and have less empty calories and still have enjoyed good calories during the week and you are maintaining your weight because you're balanced."

"Empty calories" can be in very familiar food and drinks we have every day, for example a plate of white pasta. Angelique explained how not all calories were created equal: calories have different reactions within the body. For example, if we take 500 calories as a unit of measurement for comparison, then 500 calories of white pasta will be completely different from 500 calories made up of a piece of protein with fat (fat being an integral part of protein), with vegetables, some sweet potato or brown rice. "The protein dish will give you even energy, give you your building blocks and give you the co-factors that you need to live" Angelique explained and added: "500 calories of white pasta will possibly still leave you feeling hungry because there's no nutrients in it and is going to spike your blood sugar levels within half an hour."

"Our definition of sugar needs to be expanded as well" Angelique explained: "sugar is not just the white crystallised stuff that people are no longer putting in their tea. Sugar is all the brown crystallised stuff which is actually just white sugar with molasses on, so marketing is very clever in fooling us into thinking brown sugar is better when it's clearly not."

She explained that white bread, white pasta, white flour, white sugar all become sugar (glucose) within the body really quickly. They raise our blood sugar above the level our body likes to keep us i.e. in a state of homoeostasis, a level of absolute balance. When our blood sugar levels rise, they signal for the pancreas to secrete insulin, because we can only have a certain amount of sugar within the body at any one time. This process takes the blood sugar out of the blood and into the cells, and particularly into the fat cells which make the adipose tissue.

When comparing the two 500 calories meals mentioned earlier, Angelique commented: "the difference between these two types of calories is vast. That [white pasta] would send us into low blood sugar which would stimulate hunger. On the other hand, you could have a balanced meal with protein, fats and good carbohydrates which would keep you fuller for longer. The only time I would advise you to have a bowl of white pasta with high GI, quick absorption, quick release carbohydrates is half an hour before a marathon".

There is a clear message that needs to be put out there: "Don't reward yourself with food, you're not a dog". Using food as a reward with children is particularly dangerous. Have you ever told your child: "you're being really well behaved today, so you can have an extra biscuit". "That's the wrong message" remarked Angelique, "because you now you've told her that a sweet, hydrogenated biscuit, is a 'well done, you've done really well' and that's a conditioning". We all need to rethink our relationship with food particularly with regards to "rewarding ourselves": therefore, when we need a treat, we can choose something non-food related like getting a haircut or getting a manicure (or any other "treat" of your choice). Angelique continued: "these fad diets give people a false hope that they don't have to change. All we have to do is change for a month, drop the weight, and then you don't have to be held accountable. That's quite detrimental to health or sustained good health. It's about sustainability."
The media are focusing too much on short-term weight loss but not on maintaining health.

To achieve balance we need to understand the 80/20 concept: when we have a balanced lifestyle we can afford, for example, to go to a party and have one piece a cake or 1-2 alcoholic drinks, as long as you haven't had 5 pieces of cake during the week or alcohol each night.
One slice of cake is not going to cause chronic disease, but once slice of cake three times a day is. Being honest with your friends and getting them on your side when you are aiming to lose weight makes a difference. Share you health goals with them and ask them to support you along the way.
More from Angelique: "It's not about being heroes: it's about being more present, being more aware. You have a choice what your old age is going to be like. The heroic message is: I want to live healthy and not be ill, so I am going to do this for me. If we can get people to say that, it might help. It's not a diet, it's a way of life.

Looking at what fits with your life with the guidelines on what is optimal health, what do we need to do to be really healthy."

## A Word on "Superfoods"

"Superfoods": yes, no, maybe? When I asked Angelique about super foods, her reply was: "if the research is there, and if a culture has been using it for centuries, then yes. Maca powder has been used for fertility for centuries. If we look at the properties of blueberries they have an antioxidant effect on the body. Do I think you should only have a cup of "superfoods" powders to replace food? No. They should be an addition to your well-balanced meals."

Talking of "superfoods", it is worth checking where they come from and how they are grown: do they come from a reputable company? Are they grown organically? It is worth paying a bit more and have quality assurance. Let's not forget that even "superfoods" can be sinful, as in the case of goji berries, for example, they are high in fructose. "It's all about balance", Angelique reminds us: "getting the right fat, protein, carbohydrates, fibre, hydration daily at every meal".

Look at your plate and ask yourself: is it going to heal me or is it going to harm me? If the answer is, 'it's going to harm me', what can I change in it right now that is going to have more healing properties? If you are having a bowl of white pasta, you can add dark leafy vegetables, add some fats to it to slow down the quick energy release.

## Keeping Emotions outside the Dining Room

We talked earlier about food and reward, as well as hunger and boredom. Do you tend to reach for a bar of chocolate when you are down or hand something sweet to your child as a reward? These types of associations create an artificial relationship with food. Also, could guilt be making you fat?

Do you need to lose weight? Do you want to lose weight? What are the motivations for losing weight? How much is your need to lose weight dictated by what other people think of you or pressures from the media?

When it comes to dieting, guilt could be playing a major role. Emotions run high – as babies and children, we may have been rewarded with food for good behaviour.

The key to successful weight loss is to separate emotions from the mechanical act of meal planning, cooking and eating. Consider these three mechanical activities related to food as merely part of your daily routine; remembering that, ultimately, food is simply fuel.

For example, if you are bored, do you go to the kitchen and open the fridge, almost in hope of finding some "entertainment" from food?

Boredom can be the worst enemy when starting a new healthy eating regime.

## Regimes Restricting Foods: Orthorexia and Veganism

Feelings of control could lead to extreme eating behaviours. Orthorexia is very real – it is an obsessive behaviour when only foods considered as "healthy" are allowed. It can be quite common in the well-being industry and it can lead to skipping meals, as nothing is "worthy" if it is not organic and natural. Veganism tends to restrict the types of foods that are allowed and it can have its risks. Angelique is very familiar with both eating behaviours orthorexia and veganism, as she has not only seen them in her clients but experienced them herself: "I am very aware, I have seen the signs. The reasons for people to become vegan are really important for me – when we follow a vegan diet the B12 can be lacking. Iron we get from meat is better absorbed than the iron we get from vegetable sources, and the Omega properties are better absorbed from fish oils." She recommends to be a "smart vegan" and take the right supplements to avoid vitamin and mineral deficiencies. Being vegan does not make one immune from chronic disease if the diet lacks variety: "the food diaries of some of my vegan clients" Angelique explained, "may have white flour for breakfast, white pasta for lunch and potatoes for dinner – there's no protein in that. The time when I was at my most ill was when I was vegan because I was an unhealthy vegan, which led me into my own personal eating disorder journey, but I recognised it. When I think back, I didn't have any pulses, I hardly had any dark leafy vegetables, I didn't take any supplementation and I think as a vegan we must make sure we get our B vitamins, getting our iron levels tested regularly, getting our Vitamin D tested regularly and making sure that our fatty acids status is up to date because those are very important for optimum health". Fertility is also affected, both for women and men, when there is a B vitamin deficiency "there's so many pathways that rely on B vitamins, especially vitamin B12. Being a smart vegan is essential" Angelique explained and concluded by saying "there are religious cultures that have been vegan for centuries. My message is: fat doesn't make you fat, sugar does. And sugar is the wrinkle monster." I also recommended reading Angelique's brave article on her personal journey: Eating disorders, hypothyroidism, PCOS, fertility, conception & miscarriage.

## Tips:

- Studies revealed that soups are more filling than dry food. The process of blending food means that any water that is mixed with food will stay in the stomach for longer
- ensure you have healthy foods available in the office or when you are on the go
- avoid "empty calories" as much as possible and have alcohol-free nights most of the week

# 3 Walking for Good Health

I interviewed Diet & Movement Specialist Joanna Hall, who, like me, is a firm believer in the benefits of walking for overall health and weight/inch loss. Not only I am a firm believer in walking as a great form of exercise, but I am also the proud owner of a firm bottom and I credit daily walking for this achievement.

To gain the maximum health and fitness benefits from walking, though, you need to put in some work. A leisurely stroll it isn't.

Joanna devised a walking technique called 'Walkactive' which engages all the muscles in the body while constantly correcting and improving your posture.

Twenty minutes walking using this technique feel like an hour of normal walking, which means you are making the most out of your "walk-out" (walking workout). More on that later on.

Time, many people lament, is never enough. From work commitments taking over most of the day, to social and family commitments taking most of the evenings and weekends, there isn't any time left to walk. Or is there?

## Health Benefits of Walking

Walking has been attracting more attention in the media in recent years because of its health benefits.

According to the American Heart Association, regular exercise including walking can help lower blood pressure and increase levels of good cholesterol.

Studies have reported that daily walking can be beneficial in reducing the risk of developing Alzheimer's disease.

The World Health Organisation published a report in association with Europe Health Economic Assessment Tool (HEAT).

The great news is that walking a mile a day can cut risk of dying from cancer by 40%.

The study reports that both prostate cancer and breast cancer suffers can enjoy a reduction in unpleasant side effects and mortality rate by walking at least 20 minutes a day.

Celebrity advocates of walking include musician and producer Nile Rodgers, who was stricken by prostate cancer in 2010: he credited walking as beneficial during recovery and a way to stay healthy.

Huffington Post founder Arianna Huffington has praised the benefits of walking in her book Thrive.

UK broadcaster Clare Balding dedicated a book to walking: Walking Home.

Make Google Maps your best friend and start planning and thinking up new walking routes.

## Why Buy Food when You can Forage it (and Walk at the same time)?

There's more to walking than just exercise. As a species we stopped being hunter-gatherers for survival about 10,000 years ago but this should not mean that farming should be mutually exclusive with foraging.

Intensive farming may be to blame for the lack of variety in our diet and our over-reliance on simple carbohydrates. We can add more variety to our food by going foraging for wild foods, which are rich in nutrients.

You will be surprised at how many edible plants there are out there – you just need to do your homework and, of course, go on some long, meandering walks.

Those of you who live in London can look up foraging groups and guided walks to learn more about foraging; a good starting point is the website Forage London, founded by John Rensten. John compares foraging to "a quiet, careful, sense stimulating treasure hunt".

John Rensten talked to me about urban foraging: the following is an extract of our conversation. From being a commercial photographer via a stint as a co-founder of a gastropub, John took to foraging in the early 2000s.

We started the interview talking about wild foods and their properties: wild foods, in fact, have unusually high proportions of vitamins, minerals and antioxidants plus phytonutrients, those compounds that make plants bitter and are designed to protect them from UV light, toxicity, fungi and diseases.

"There's a lot of people who say "I want to do a paleolithic diet" and just eat meat and vegetables but the paleo vegetables that has been around would have been small and massively fibrous and very bitter. So if you go on a paleolithic diet and eat meat and sweetcorn – sweetcorn now is the equivalent of a Mars Bar. When I tried to do my blog about 'superfoods' I couldn't because all wild foods are 'superfoods'."

Introducing some wild foods in your diet can be good for your health: rose hip, for example, has 20 times the amount of vitamin C compared to oranges, weight by weight. Crab apples contain malic acid which can be beneficial to combat chronic fatigue and remove heavy metals from the body.

You don't need to live in the countryside to enjoy the great outdoors and benefit from wild foods.

A walk to your local woods and local parks can be very fruitful, just not the royal parks, as manicured lawns are pretty pointless for this exercise. Your local park may surprise you with unexpected goodies. I would suggest you look up local guides who can teach you about edible plants that grow spontaneously. You can also join local walking groups of foragers.

Free food anyone?

Well, not quite. Check your local legislation on what you are allowed to pick. For example, in London you need permission to dig up roots, and you need to be aware that parks are not common land but private property that we are granted access to.

Talking of London: did you know that 47% of London is made of green space? Of this percentage, 60% is open space (the rest is allotments and private gardens).

With 8 million trees, London is one of the world's largest urban forests. In the UK there are 15 national parks. To make Londoners more aware of how much green space there is, Dave Raven-Ellison walked 75 km across London in one day from Croydon in the South to Barnet in the North.

Most people live in an urban environment. "There's 6 million people in London and in the middle of the daytime it is 18 million people", John explained, "that's a third of the entire population of the whole country in Central London. That is dense. Very frenetic and very toxic on numerous different levels."

John described his own journey into foraging as follows: "my city goggles switched off, and on came my wild food vision" and continued: "I've set up Forage London to give city dwellers like myself a chance to enjoy and discover some of the amazing wild foods that grow all around us."

We are consuming too much and we are not too aware of how our food choices affect the environment. To John, grazing is the answer: "sampling numerous plants, herbs, wild foods, but mostly in very small amounts, experiencing new flavours and learning how these change with the seasons with a view to getting out of the city more".

He doesn't like to call himself an "expert" but simply someone who takes people on a walk and shows them how to observe and learn about their environment. You learn by looking, touching, smelling, tasting (what John calls "informed nibbling") and that is a multi-sensory way of learning that not only is more stimulating than sitting in a class, but also the information you gather is more likely to stay in your long term memory. We mentioned earlier on the way Ancient Greeks used to impart knowledge by going out walking... they were obviously ahead of time.

There is so much biodiversity even in urban parks, if you know where to look. You need to be very selective, though, in terms of what you pick and where you pick food for foraging, because pollution levels can be high.

Most London parks (or other urban parks) could be hosting more than 100 types of edible plants.

John explained that there are two main groups of plants:

wild plants that are hardy, robust and don't need to be fertilised and could reclaim the city within 15 years if we all disappeared because they thrive on neglect; some of these plants have medicinal properties trees and plants that have been planted intentionally by town and park planners, and within this group some plants are edible

Urban environments are quite different from rural ones: sometimes there's extended seasons as winters are milder in built-up areas so plants stay in flower longer.

The bigger the urban environment, the bigger the micro-climate. There's a far greater overlapping of seasons, there's an increase in fertility, and things stay in flower longer. You find that plants' seasons elongated.

"I wanted to explore London and I researched the parks" John explained, "I found that I could run walks, I backed up my knowledge with some far more academic study than I had previously needed and then I started running walks and they have been really successful."

A word of warning: "When I take people on walks in an urban environment I don't advocate that they descend upon their local green space and try to turn it into a source of sustainable food. I'm quite specific about this because it's easy to get confused to think you are on common land when you are not on common land. You're on private property. If you want to do something in that environment you've got to obey the rules or, if you're going to twist or abuse the rules, you need to do it with a certain amount of respect or subtlety." In addition to which, there are discussions to be had about toxicity and pollution.

When choosing where to walk always look for green spaces away from the traffic and that are not accessible to dogs as dog waste is particularly toxic.

You also must remember that foraging in urban environments is not a "free for all" and does not replace your trip to the supermarket: you are allowed to pick foodstuff in small amounts but you should be responsible and considerate, respecting property (urban parks are usually owned by local councils).

"When I take people on walks in an urban environment I don't advocate that they descend upon their local green space and try to turn it into a source of sustainable food" John pointed out. "I'm quite specific about this because it's easy to get confused to think you are on common land when you are not on common land" he continued.

You also need to be aware of the toxicity of plants and not pick something you don't recognise, which is why it is always advisable to learn foraging with a guide and do plenty of research first.

John said "When I'm in a city I don't eat a lot of wild food, I nibble a little bit, but when I'm out of the city my fridge just fills up, I don't try it just does. I leave the house and come back with food. What I tend to do I nibble bits so use it more like an educational tool."

"We come to the concept of toxicity because I'm sure in my wanderings I ingest the odd bit of dog wee and it doesn't do me any harm but, having said that, toxicaria canis (that is, the little bug that gets on dog poo) can cause blindness and liver flu (little worm that lives on some water plants can attack your liver) can make you really ill."

John runs walks in Dorset and the New Forest for those city dwellers who want to explore the countryside. He also runs walks for charities like Blue Ventures.

A lot of things that we pick are poisonous raw and edible when cooked. You have to use a lot of common sense. Misidentifying things can be dangerous – John is particularly aware of this and has dedicated a section of his website on sensible foraging. "My feeling is that if you live in London you sign on for a degree of toxicity. It's not just toxicity in terms of traffic – it's toxicity in terms of mobile phones, drinking too much coffee, people's attitudes, drink/drug culture. How munching a few plants in your local parks does or does not contribute to that toxicity I generally suggest people do their own research" John commented, and added "I make a lot of remedies myself". In his walks he talks about medicine, herbalism, nutrition, local history.

## The Culture of Foraging

John compares foraging to a treasure hunt and the process of learning about foraging as the antidote to our frenetic lives: "nature gives up its secrets gradually. You learn in a slow way it's the opposite of the internet: you come back and you gradually get you the information that you need over time."

You look at how things change and it gets you in contact with the seasons and even more than that it's far more than seasonal, it's more time-specific. Things change in a week or in a day, flavours change as well. You may taste something one day and it becomes pollinated and the next day it's delicious, or vice-versa.

"A lot of foraging it's not about what you pick but it's about what you do with what you pick. Sometimes an hour foraging will lead to four hours in the kitchen" John enthused; "everybody can go out and forage pretty much immediately because everybody knows what a stinging nettle looks like, it is a fantastic foraging plant."

Stinging nettle is a perennial plant so you can go back to it for new growth. Some stinging nettle varieties come out with leaves as big as dinner plates. In mid summer you can even tempura them: dip them in batter and fry for a delicious starter or side dish. In March time you can sweat stinging nettle in a little oil like you would do with spinach or use it in a curry. In September you get nettle seeds and you can cook with them. They have a high protein content and are also a stimulant. As you can see there's a numerous ways you can use stinging nettle during the year.

With elderflower and elderberry you need to learn about it properly and do your research to ensure you don't confuse it with dogwood flowers. Both elderflower and dogwood bloom in May; dogwood flowers in sprays at about the same time in the year and looks similar to elderflower. In late summer the elder plant produces berries: you can caper green berries by storing them in salt for about three weeks and then you pickle them. When the elder berries are mature you can use them to make jam, vinegar or cordial. As you can see, from the same plant you get different crops spread over a few months. Other examples include wild garlic, which gives five crops in 2-3 months, and lime trees with three crops spread across the year.

Another good foraging plant is dandelion: you've got flowers you can make wine and jam with. You can make vinegar with the flowers. Dandelion leaves available all year round. They are a bit bitter but you can force them, i.e., you can blanch them by putting a pot over them so they grow in the dark. You can also use the dandelion root, which has a really nice tender texture and you can fry, boil or roast it. Roast dandelion root has been used for years as a coffee substitute. Once again, you get many different uses from the same plant across the year.

Mallow and chickweed are good foraging plant being very easy to identify once you have been shown them. Both produce multiple crops.

The lime tree (or linden or tilia) is a brilliant foraging plant. First of all, it is a calmative; it also produces 3 crops. The leaves are full of mucilage, the same gelatinous substance you would find in okra, which helps the digestive transit. They are good to eat in salads. Because the leaves shoot from the trunk you get a lot of new growth, so you could potentially be picking these leaves for 4-5 months.

You then get the blossoms which you can eat straight off the tree and they smell and taste like honeydew melon. You can use them for cordials and syrups. John explained: "I made a lime blossom champagne and it's wonderful. It tastes like a slightly fruity champagne and with almost like a flavour of tea, almost like an iced tea." But there's more: "then you also have the unopened leaf buds which you get in winter which are small and red and the tree is easy to recognise then because the shoots come off from the trunk and you can put the red buds in salads. That's a brilliant urban plant."

Elderberries contain high levels of vitamin C and have antibacterial properties.

Hawthorn is another good plant with plenty of healing properties – just like the lime tree, young hawthorn leaves can be used in salads.

## A lovely Way to Learn

John's message is "go foraging because it's good for you: it's good for your brain to absorb information in a slow way instead of such a fast way. It's multi-sensory: it involves your brain, your eyes, your memory, your nose, your sense of touch, your recognition. It gets you outside. You look at something, you then go look in a book, you look at it again, you might pick it, you may watch it change as the seasons change, see it in different states, you may cook it or turn it into something, use it in a different ways. It's a lovely way to learn. I'm stunned at how much I retained. I never was like that at school."

Of course, food safety always comes first: "I make a lot of home remedies myself. You should be careful with contraindications. On a walk I talk about medicine, herbalism, cookery, horticulture, nutrition, foraging, local history. And I feed people lots of bits." John uses nibbling as an educational tool to reinforce learning (a multi-sensory experience).

The recommendation is to have a consultation with a professionally qualified herbalist before taking (or making your own) herbal remedies. Some herbs can be toxic and all herbal medicine preparations sold by suppliers must go through strict quality controls.

Then there's the whole concept of "superfoods": if you look at what is described as a "superfood" it has unusually high proportion of vitamins, minerals, nutrients, antioxidants. Wild foods have that, plus phytonutrients which make plants taste bitter. John explained: "phytonutrients are chemical compounds that are in the plant and are designed to be there to protect it from UV, from us, from toxicity, from animals, from various diseases, from fungi. 400 generations of farming have mostly bred out all of the things in our food chain that was good for us and replaced it with carbohydrates i.e., sugar."

We mentioned the "paleo" diet before – I wanted to ask John what he thought about it: "there's a lot of people who say 'I want to do a paleolithic diet' and just eat meat and vegetables but the paleo vegetables that has been around would have been small and massively fibrous and very bitter." So if you go on a true paleolithic diet today and, for example, you eat meat and sweetcorn, you are ingesting protein, but with a high level of sugar, because "sweetcorn now is the equivalent of a Mars Bar. When I tried to do my blog about superfood I couldn't because all wild foods are superfoods." The idea of an apple a day doesn't keep the doctor away any more – John explained: "it's about 28 apples you need nowadays and alas you'd be ingesting so much sugar in the process".

John continued: "I'm not advocating that everybody stops working and start foraging but if you introduce a little bit of foraged food in your diet it will help you: it will help your health."

Most of the phytonutrients are extremely good for you, however not all of them are and you need to be aware of that. Phytonutrients are there to help the plant in numerous ways. Rose hip is a good example. Rose hips, weight for weight, have 20 times more vitamin C than oranges and contain masses of antioxidants and pectin which is excellent for supporting your liver if you have a detox. Talking of detoxification, another good crop is the crab apple, which contains malic acid. Malic acid is excellent in helping remove heavy metals from your body.

So what is John's opinion of supermarkets? "I'm not anti supermarkets because big cities and monoculture go hand in hand and at the moment we have cities and we have mono-cultures and we have supermarkets. I'm not saying let's all go foraging because that is silly. I find it unpleasant that, say, if you've got 95 products that are all bad for you and 5 that are called 'superfoods' and are good for you but are very expensive. I can't quite see the logic to where we have arrived."

**Foraging for Beginners**

First of all, do your research. Good books to start with include:

- Neil Fletcher's The Easy Wild Food Guide,
- John Wright's Hedgerow,
- Roger Phillips' Wild Food,
- Richard Mabey's Food for Free

John said: "foraging is absolutely easy. Find somebody who is running walks, it's invaluable. You learn far more that way than you would any other way. I've got a blog on my website about how to identify all members of the mint family 50 plants in 10 minutes. If you learn 50 plants in 10 minutes (and I can teach you those 50 plants in 10 minutes right now,) in that whole mint family there's only one you need to avoid. It's very easy to find the one you need to avoid, because it looks very different, and then you've got 50 plants that you can go foraging for."

Everybody can go out and forage pretty much immediately because everybody knows what a stinging nettle looks like, it is a fantastic foraging plant.

Are you mad about mushrooms? I am. Again, with mushrooms in particular the message is safety first, as there are some varieties which are lethal when ingested (either raw or cooked). Some relatively safe mushrooms can cause food poisoning when eaten raw, and remember that cooking does not make poisonous mushrooms edible. John explained that there's about 12 different wild mushrooms that you can learn easily. However, you still need to be very careful and always go out on your first mushroom foraging walks with an experienced guide "to help you sort the delicious from the deadly" as John said on his website. The safest mushrooms which are edible are the giant puffball (which looks like a football) and the hedgehog mushroom (which, instead of having gills, has spines). John warned: "I don't advocate foraging for mushrooms in an urban environment because of the toxicity of the environment, which they are fantastic at absorbing."

| Plant | When to pick |
|---|---|
| Crab apple | From autumn but plenty of windfalls right through January |
| Dandelion | Leaves and flowers most of the year and roots best picked early spring or late autumn |
| Wild Garlic | Starts in March in London, later in other parts. Edible parts are leaves, shoots, bulbs, flowers and seeds |
| Stinging Nettle | Young growth in the spring time, new growth later in the year too |
| Elder | Flowers around May and berries in September |
| Lime | Leaves much earlier but delicious blossoms start around June |
| Cherry | June and July, also sweet blossoms before |
| Blackberries | September, sometimes much earlier |
| Hazel | Ideally earlier to avoid the squirrels but ripe around October. Better eaten green earlier |
| Sloes | Ideally with the first frost but often earlier |
| Rose hips, Rosa rugosa | Some types in August, while other types right through to mid winter |
| Mahonia | Sweet yellow flowers in December and purple berries earlier in the year |

John's tips for foraging beginners are:

- if you are going to pick any plant work out how high a dog will cock his leg and don't pick below that although dog wee is very acidic so you will see the leaves looking burnt, not healthy

- stay away from the roads and polluted areas
- don't eat urban fungi
- don't turn anything that you find into a source of food for a protracted period of time. Pick something here and there.
- do a little bit of research about where you are foraging. It may look like a beautiful green space that has been there for years but you may find out in the 20s there was a bomb factory there which is a really classic example.

For example, say you pick wild spinach from a cemetery: you may find out the spinach has been growing on lead and arsenic. "I avoid cemeteries completely" John said.

On one side, cemeteries have been green spaces for a long time; on the flip side, there's an awful lot of arsenic that has been used in our cemeteries, and lead.

Additionally, try not to dwell in the same spot, but move around and look for different foraging spots to ensure you are less exposed to toxicity.

**Walking Activities**

You will hit a wall at one point when you will start becoming bored of walking, even after changing your scenic routes.

You can mix things up by combining walking with other activities. Foraging, as mentioned before, is an option: if foraging with a group, it can become a social activity. Foraging also makes you look at your surroundings differently, as you take in more of what's around you.

Related to walking and foraging is urban gardening and guerrilla gardening: for example, Future Green Studio in New York organises walks to identify and categorise spontaneous plants and create green spaces in highly developed areas. Activities like this can be great not only for socialising but also for learning about plants.

Other activities include walking tours – check with your local tour guides. In London, for example, you can join walking tours and learn about history, architecture, literature, cinema.

If you are a member of a book club, you could organise a book walk and talk (London once again has book walks like the ones organised by the Society of Young Publishers).

Whether you live in London or you are just visiting it, I recommend a guided walk in Highgate Wood. The calendar of events for guided walks include history, wildlife, herbalism, mushrooms, insects and even bat watching.

I attended a guided walk about history, conservation, and arborism. You absorb so much information as you walk, as you reinforce your learning by observing and listening. Our walking group learned about conservation areas, that allow birds to nest, and wildlife and wild plants to thrive.

Covering 28 hectares of woodland, and keeping the site for public enjoyment since 1886, Highgate Wood won the Green Heritage Award for managing sites of historic importance. It is possible that the woods have been used since Roman times as pottery shards were discovered there.

## Green Tourism

You can take walking to the next level and carefully choose holidays with the lowest impact on the environment.

Walking holidays are the perfect example, but how much carbon emission will you need to offset if you are travelling by plane?

An alternative is to travel within your country by public transport and take any opportunity to cover some distance walking or cycling.

The next step is to check the environmental credentials of the places you will be staying at.

Hotels tend to be more wasteful in terms of water usage, for example: just the laundry has a great impact on the environment. Waste water is an issue too.

Some venues take the treatment of waste water very seriously and they will happily provide any documentation to show how green they are (you can, for example, check for any environmental awards they have won).

You could check if the holiday venue has solar panels, plenty of recycling collection points for plastic, paper, glass and batteries.

You can use the holiday as an opportunity to observe the wildlife and wild flowers – and, why not, go foraging.

Camping may not be everybody's cup of tea, but there are camping holidays that provide more comfort than the average by providing luxury cabins and lodges. I stayed in a spotless and sparkling leisure lodge within Oakdown Holiday Park in East Devon once and it did not feel like camping at all. I had my own kitchen and bathroom and one of the most comfortable beds I have ever slept in. Owner Doreen Franks went out of her way to make me feel comfortable and explain more about the local attractions like Beer Quarry caves where limestone had been mined since Roman times. That's just one example of alternative holidays – you can be a discerning customer and choose accordingly.

**Awareness and Mindfulness**

Alongside the health benefits of walking as a form of exercise, there are added bonus features that can help you with losing weight and keeping it off.

Instead of obsessing over food or a specific body part (or cellulite), start a daily practice of scanning your body for areas of tension, or simply become more familiar with your own body. Does it feel flexible? Hot? Cold? Each subtle sign can say plenty about your state of health.

To me walking gives me an opportunity to ground myself, feel more relaxed, more balanced: walking as an opportunity to have a mind/body connection in a dynamic way. I asked Sophrologist Dominique Antiglio of BeSophro to explain how we can integrate dynamic relaxation and meditation in our daily life, particularly when we go out for a walk.

Personally, I found that Sophrology is an excellent way to raise mind/body awareness and is even more accessible than meditation as a form of stress management. It is also a useful tool for self-development, as you work through issues that are stopping you from achieving your goals.

While meditation is more about observation, Sophrology is more active as it allows you to influence your consciousness in a positive, non-judgemental way. In other words, you are in the driving seat and you choose how to assess your situation using your inner resources.

What is Sophrology and how can it benefit you? It is a dynamic relaxation, stress management and personal development technique. By practising Sophrology when you walk, you take the time to observe the world around you as if it was the first time. This in itself gives you freedom. Dominique explained: "you can apply it in your daily life because you have understood that by opening up the possibilities in your brain you become more creative. You can get out of your patterns. It reinforces the energy: you are walking, it's more dynamic, it's very good for the body, it's a different meditation in action, compared with just walking or being in the lotus position, it's a different way of meditating. It's learning to have stillness in action."

A lot of us are used to rushing to action. By practising Sophrology you create more time for yourself, so you avoid rushing and accomplish more. It's about learning to be present: you learn to let go of the rational mind and concentrate on what is. Dominique referred to The Power of Now author Eckhart Tolle: "(he) teaches us to be present. In Sophrology we learn to be present, we listen to sensations. Then we master the mind and then we bring mind and body together."

You can practise Sophrology while walking and it becomes meditation in action: the body and the mind are in the present moment and through movement and the intention we use is a way to know yourself better. Dominique expanded on that: "it goes beyond relaxation and feeling grounded and it can be used as a path to self-discovery. It's about entering a conscious relationship with ourselves and with what we observe around us. One of the aspects we do is opting for a non-judgemental approach to what surrounds us and to ourselves as we walk, which allows us to live things more intensely. You stop analysing what you see but you welcome the information."

For example, a simple exercise could be looking at a tree as if it was the first time: you imagine that you have never seen a tree and you don't know that green is a colour, you don't know that a tree grows and it gets bigger. You feel like a child looking at a tree for the first time.

"In Sophrology there's 12 levels of practice and we introduce walking in different levels: level 3 and 4", Dominique explained.

Sophrology is divided in 3 cycles:

cycle 1 is about calming the mind and centring yourself and being more present, letting go of what the mind doesn't need, going more in depth within and strengthening the link between mind and body

cycle 2 is about going a step further into exploring consciousness and mastering its energy

cycle 3 is about transformation and achieving greater awareness of yourself and the world around you while fine-tuning aspects of the consciousness

Walking meditation is part of the Sophrology practice – to be precise it comes in cycle 1 and in cycle 3. With walking the goal is to have an experience, to bring movement and breathing together, to increase body awareness and to bring more consciousness into action.

Walking meditation in Sophrology is inspired by Zen meditation. Eyes are semi open, you start by doing your normal seated Sophrology practice, which involves breathing, relaxation and visualisation. You will need to start with a Sophrology practitioner to understand the breathing and the exercises. Once you are in a 'sophroliminal' state (a receptive state of relaxation when you are fully aware of what is going on while being deeply relaxed) you stand up. Walking meditation is quite advanced and requires that you have already practised 3 levels of Sophrology. The easiest thing to do is to stand up, bring your fingers and arms on the hara (lower abdomen), then take some small steps. You are experimenting the change in balance, stepping to the right and to the left, like the first steps you took when you were a child. You are experimenting the walking movement as if it was the first time, observing every aspect of it as you do it.

**Walking exercise 1**

You inhale with your nose on your first 3 steps walking normally, then you hold your breath on your 4th step, you breathe out for the next 3 steps again, you hold 1 on the next step. You learn to do this as you walk, you count or you synchronise the step with a positive word, for example confidence, that you want to feel in your body. This increases oxygen in the red blood cells, it quietens the heart, it stimulates oxygenation and circulation, it allows your mind to settle and to restore, it's a very therapeutic practice and it allows presence in the here and now. It also feels blissful.

## Walking walking exercise 2: easy

This exercise requires that you have already practised Sophrology for a while (Dominique recommended from Level 4 onwards), once you have achieved a better balance of mind and body. This exercise allows you to feel more aligned to your aims and values. "Sophrology allows you to reflect on the values in your life" Dominique explained, "what are the values you hold dear in your heart? You can put your powerful mind/body energy to serve these values. For some people it's trust, for some people it's love, it's family..." The sequence of exercises that your Sophrology practitioner gives you allows you to explore your own values and find how you want to build your intention to serve these values.

In this simple walking exercise you start with your seated Sophrology practice working on your breathing, focusing on your abdomen. You then walk for 20 minutes practising a positive presence, i.e., walking as if it was the first time, exploring your surroundings without preconceived ideas. You are witnessing yourself walking in the street/park and, because you have meditated, your mindset is really clear about what you are going to do in those 20 minutes. Then you come back and sit down to continue your Sophrology practice working on your body through your breathing. Dominique explained: "it's about choosing a value, for example 'I am going to look at the world as if it was the first time, through the eyes of love for myself and for the world around me'. When you do this, because you are in the 'sophroliminal' state and you are in a deeper state of consciousness, you will be surprised at all the things that come. It's like a quest and you are getting a lot of answers during those 20 minutes, because you set a very clear intention." You will also notice that you walk slower, because you have set an intention to be mindful. You may find yourself not needing to rush so much any more. You may feel you have more time, and start noticing that people around you are walking really fast, each one of them looking so worried and preoccupied. Being open and observing the world in a state of mindfulness can be very interesting. You start noticing things you didn't see before, and events (stressful or otherwise) don't seem to affect you as much as they did before.

The good thing about a walking meditation exercise like this is that you could do it in your lunch break.

An image/device that Sophrology practitioners use to explain about the technique is Plato's Allegory of the Cave. This allegory tells the story of a group of people who are in chains and living in a cave. Each step these people take towards the exit of the cave corresponds to each step that you talk in your Sophrology journey. It's the process of freeing your consciousness from preconceived ideas and judgement. The aim is to become free human beings, who are responsible for themselves. The light at the opening of the cave in the allegory means that you look at the world differently – there' a whole wide world outside waiting to be explored. You learn to let go of the chains from the past and you start discovering new dimensions of consciousness.

## Walking exercise 3: advanced

Starting from a seated position, you stand up, inhale, tense the whole body by pressing on your lower abdomen with your hands, you exhale and relax. Then you prepare yourself for your first step by bringing your weight onto your left foot first. You bring your right foot next to the left foot by sliding it on the floor effectively taking a half step. Then you shift your body weight onto your right foot and you bring the left together with the right by sliding it on the floor. Repeat this 3 times in total and turn around. Before you take a step you inhale/tense the body and exhale/relax the body. You are preparing yourself consciously for each step that you do. Once you have turned around, you come back to your initial position by taking 3 steps and then you sit down. Do an integration pause, which means you integrate/take into account all the sensations from the experience. You are already on a path of self-discovery, bringing mind and body together and listening to the sensations from your body.

Because Sophrology is a modern technique and it not as popular in the UK or the US as it is in Spain or France, there's only a few reference books available; an example is Florence Parrot's Instant Serenity for Life and Work.

Daniel Zanin created the concept of "Conscious Walk" or "Afghan Walk" mixing Sophrology and walking. Zanin organises walks in the desert and mountains using meditation with breathing. You could use his technique as you walk in the street or in nature, for either a short or long time.

## Walking Meditation

A few years ago I attended a meditation workshop. One of the exercises was to focus on the mechanics of walking so we were asked to walk very slowly, taking time on each step and turning our attention on each micro-movement.

What we take for granted when we walk is complex interplay of synergistic movements. Without us realising it, we are using several muscles at the same time to move the body forward.

As far as the thought processes are concerned, we walk "on autopilot" so we use our autonomous nervous system to give the right commands to our muscles.

Before you set off to you next walk take the opportunity to use your problem-solving side of the brain and take it for a spin. Set the purpose of the walk as you set off: you may have a question or a problem that are still unresolved. Once you have started your walk forget about the question and simply walk taking in the surroundings and noticing how your feet make contact with the ground. Feel the breeze on your face; feel the movement in your arms and in your legs. It's easy to get lost in the walk - not literally but metaphorically. Let go of the problems that are worrying you and allow your mind to rest. Keep on walking and try make your walk to last at least an hour for full benefits.

The key is not to obsess over the problem but to release it as if you are letting go of a helium balloon floating away from your hand.

You can also use the time of your walk to explore any feelings you have about your body and notice any areas of tension. A walking meditation is a way to reconnect with your inner self and there's no need to sit in the yoga lotus position to achieve a sense of inner calm.

You may want to use your daily walks as a generic stress management tool: replace worrying and with walking.

Worrying requires plenty of mental energy that could be better deployed elsewhere, for example to set goals and make plans to achieve them.

Worry will put your whole body on high alert and triggers the release of stress hormones: that's when the "fight or flight" mechanism kicks in.

When we are stressed and worried we end up seeing things in tunnel vision instead of seeing the whole picture, as Mark Williams explained during a talk at the School of Life. That's a similar analogy to the Allegory of the Cave mentioned earlier.

I say put your brain to good use: let your brain's creative juices marinade any worries, negative thoughts and feelings, and grill those nasties to make a tasty snack!

If we look at the Buddhist tradition, walking meditations are done mostly alone, at times in a group.

There's no right or wrong way to do a walking meditation, but if you wanted to follow the Buddhist tradition you could start with a simple 20 minute walk, on a very slow pace. Plan those 20 minutes carefully so you don't get interrupted: switch off your phone and leave the errands to later. You may want to start your walking meditation by standing still and concentrating on your breathing. After three in breaths and out breaths, start breathing normally and begin your walk.

To achieve a meditative state, choose a quiet place where you can walk backwards and forwards undisturbed. Start by walking at a very slow pace, to allow your mind to rest. After 15 minutes, walk even slower, letting go of all worries. After another 15 minutes, walk at a moderate pace but still slow enough. Always set your intention before you start walking: your intention could be that you want to practice stillness and mindfulness.

As you slow down, notice the movement of your foot lifting off the ground then gently making contact with the ground walking forward. You may also want to count the steps from 1 to 10 and then back to 1 again.

You will be tempted to count beyond 10 so if you catch yourself mentally counting 11, simply go back to 1 and start again. You may want to breathe in when you take your first step and breathe out when you take the next step. There's a "do it yourself" walking meditation guide on Wikipedia.

I found this quote from Insight Meditation Center in California quite useful: "traditional Buddhist teachings identify four meditation postures: sitting, walking, standing and lying down. All four are valid means of cultivating a calm and clear mindfulness of the present moment. The most common meditation posture after sitting is walking. In meditation centres and monasteries, indoor halls and outdoor paths are often built for walking meditation. On meditation retreats, regular walking meditation is an integral part of the schedule. In practice outside of retreats, some people will include walking as part of their daily meditation practice".

Walking Technique

The way we walk makes all the difference to get the maximum health and weight loss results from this cardiovascular activity.

From posture to foot positioning, walking can be tweaked and perfected for optimum performance.

I would recommend using Joanna Hall's Walkactive guidelines.

The key components of a good walking techniques are:

- the feet
- the hips
- the core (abdominal muscles)
- the shoulders
- the arms

If you can, ask a friend or your partner to video you while you walk: how is your posture? Do you slouch? Do you shuffle your feet or do you make contact with the floor with the heel first, then the sole and then the ball of your feet and your toes?

Do you keep your abdominal muscles tight or do you allow your belly to flop?

Using the body the way it was designed to move can not only allow you to improve the way you walk but in the long term it can prevent injuries and slow down the inevitable wear and tear on the joints as we age.

As a welcome side effect, walking tall and with the correct technique can contribute to lift your moods and your overall well-being.

Walkactive is a scientifically proven effective walking system created by Joanna Hall. Let's hear from Joanna herself, who kindly shared her knowledge and experience.

"'Walkactive' was independently validated by South Bank University Sports Performance Laboratory. 'Walkactive' has been

scientifically proven to be more effective than normal working.
It is statistically proven to:

- trim the waist line
- anti-age posture
- reduce joint stress
- lose weight

compared to normal working." In the article "Walk this way for fitness" it was reported that, after 28 days, 3% reduction in body fat and 15% reduction in waist measurement.

Joanna explained: "the system relates to a simple 4 part process so the body walks with correct postural & the body achieves a streamlined toned shape through the muscles working through a lengthened tautening effect. Training the body from the inside to stimulate the fascia – the workout sessions are deceptively gentle but highly effective."

Specific health benefits to Walkactive include:

significant reduction in joint discomfort.

posture improvement

reduction in anti depressant medication

reduction in statin medication

reduction in blood pressure

positive contribution in operation recovery specifically.

Joanna added: "mastering the 'Walkactive' System creates a smooth flowing anti ageing movement quality which creates fluid effortless motion.

Once mastered, the Walkactive System fits easily into a busy life so it's perfect for time short individuals as well as exercise fanatics who wish to take their walking workouts to the next level for total body improvement & confidence. For more information on the Walkactive System, audio coaching sessions & videos please visit www.joannahall.com".

**Tips:**

Here's a handy list of things you should look out for when you're walking to make sure you are getting a good cardiovascular workout:

- aim to walk at a slightly faster pace than normal – you should be able to still hold a conversation but feel slightly out of breath

- you should feel that the back of your legs are working, not just the front
- you should feel that your glutes are working – normally your bottom does not get enough exercise, especially if you have a sedentary job
- allow your shoulders to move away from your ears and lengthen your neck
- try not to clench your jaw as you walk to avoid neck pain – when we are stressed we clench muscles without realising
- use your arms to give you more momentum

## And finally... one more Reason to Love Walking

I asked sex and relationship expert Tracey Cox what her thoughts were on the benefits of walking: in a nutshell, you can walk your walk to a better libido.

"• Exercise is linked with boosting your sex drive. Most people feel more energized after exercise and good about themselves and their body. Walking is one of the best exercises around and keeps your mood nice and elevated for hours afterwards, which means you'll be brilliant company over dinner – and still have energy afterwards for a romp around the bedroom.

• The fitter you are physically, the higher your sex drive and the more often you'll want to have sex. If you're unfit, you're lethargic. Everything is an effort and you tire easily so the fitter you are, the longer your sex sessions usually are.

• Fitter people who walk often instigate sex more often and last longer when they do. They like their bodies more – if you like your body, you want to show it off."

Walking holidays or other walking activity to do together can help strengthen a relationship. For example, walking side by side allows for better conversation, as there's less eye contact and you can explore issues that hadn't been talked about before.

# 4 Healthy recipes

### Gluten-free and dairy-free Strawberry Pancakes
Ingredients:
4 medium strawberries
3 tablespoons gluten-free flour
1 medium organic egg
1 tablespoon oil
ground cinnamon or vanilla sugar optional
Method:
In a blender blitz the egg and flour together, then add the strawberries. Mix until there's no clumps.
Heat a shallow non-stick pan then add half of the oil for the first batch of pancakes (approximately 5 small pancakes).
Pour the pancake mixture in the pan with a spoon (1 spoonful per pancake), cook for 2-3 minutes and flip over cooking a further 2-3 minutes.
Serve immediately with a dusting of cinnamon or vanilla sugar.
Another option is to make crepes instead and fill them with chopped fresh fruit or chocolate spread.

### Spelt Risotto with Butternut Squash
Ingredients:
50 gr butternut squash, chopped
50 gr sweet potato, chopped
50 gr onion, chopped (frozen is fine)
70 gr spelt
30 gr truffle pesto (or normal pesto)
1/2 tablespoon vegetable bouillon
1/2 litre water
Method:
In a large pan, cook the chopped sweet potato and butternut squash with the onion and a bit of water. Let the ingredients become softer (3-5 minutes) then add the rest of the water, vegetable bouillon and the spelt.
Cook for 10-15 minutes at a medium heat, stirring every few

minutes. When the spelt is cooked through, turn off the heat and add the pesto.

To speed up the prep time, use ready chopped sweet potato, butternut squash and onions.

## Guam Chopped Chicken and Coconut Salad
Ingredients:
1 boneless chicken leg
1 onion
2 tablespoons soy sauce
2 tablespoons cider vinegar
1 teaspoon ground black pepper
60 grams fresh grated coconut
2 Thai chillies
Juice of 1 lemon
1 glass water for the marinade
1 bunch mixed fresh herbs (oregano, thyme, mint and lemon balm; original recipe requires green onions)
1 chapatti (or pitta bread)
Method:
Marinade the boneless chicken leg the night before with the onion (sliced), soy sauce, vinegar, pepper and water. Put in an air-tight container and store in the fridge.

Remove the chicken from the marinade and drain well (you can use the marinade as a base for gravy or other sauce). Cook under the grill for 25-30 minutes or until cook through, turning over to ensure both sides are cooked (original recipe says to cook over a barbecue for approximately 30 minutes) or in the oven.

Serve the salad cold: you need to cool down the chicken, cut it into small cubes and combine it to fresh grated coconut, chillies, chopped fresh herbs and lemon juice.

Serve with a warmed chapatti (or pitta bread). You can substitute the green onions from the traditional recipe with fresh herbs and the chicken with Quorn.

## Summer Salad Recipe: Cherries, Cherry Tomatoes, Avocado and Green Beans
Ingredients:
50 gr green beans
10 cherries
4 cherry tomatoes
1 avocado
1 tablespoon olive oil

1 teaspoon cider vinegar

Optional: sunflower or pumpkin seeds for extra crunch and protein

Method:

Boil or steam the green beans for 3-5 minutes so they remain crunchy. Add the beans to a bowl with the cherry tomatoes cut in half, the cherries also halved and with the stone removed, 1 sliced avocado and the dressing made of olive oil and cider vinegar. Mix well and serve immediately.

## Quick Apricot "Tarte Tatin" (gluten and dairy free)

Ingredients:

5 apricots

1 egg

100 grams gluten free self-raising flour (I used a blend of rice, potato, maize, tapioca and buckwheat)

2 tablespoons olive oil

100 grams soya milk

50 grams sugar (Demerara/cane sugar)

Method:

Melt the sugar in a pan with a little water; when it turns golden, add the apricots, washed and cut in half. Cook the apricots until they are soft, turning over a couple of times. Depending on the size of the apricots, cook for about 5 minutes; they should still be a bit firm and not mushy. For a nicer presentation, have them skin side down in the pan. Add 1 tablespoon of oil.

Mix the egg, flour, 1 tablespoon olive oil and milk with a whisk and pour the pancake mixture into the pan with the apricots and sugar syrup.

Cook for approximately 3 minutes, then move over to a heated grill and crisp up the top for a further 3 minutes. Use a toothpick to check that the batter is completely cooked through, then serve flipping the pan over to reveal the apricots topping.

## Fruity Duck Salad

Ingredients:

10 gr Fresh spinach

20 gr Mixed salad leaves

30 gr Kale

1 Avocado

1 duck breast
1 mango
1 slice watermelon (100 gr)
20 gr roasted cashew nuts
1 small piece of fresh ginger, grated
2 tablespoons soy sauce
1 lime
½ teaspoon Himalayan salt (or table salt)
1 Thai red chilli
Method:
Roast the duck breast in the oven (220 degrees Celsius) for 20 minutes or until the skin is crispy and the meat is cooked through. Place the duck skin side up on a roasting tray and just sprinkle with a pinch of salt, no oil required.

Tear off the kale leaves into small pieces and discard the stalks (you can freeze the stalks and use them in soups). "Massage" the kale with a bit of olive oil, salt and half the juice of a lime. Squeeze and crunch the kale with your hands until it gets darker in colour.

To assemble the salad: chop the watermelon, mango and avocado into small cubes; add the kale, fresh leaves and roasted cashews.

For the salad dressing: slice the chilli and add to a pan with the soy sauce, remaining lime juice and grated ginger. Warm up for two minutes, then drizzle over the salad.

## Mini Burgers with Brussels Sprouts
Ingredients:
8 Brussels sprouts
16 thin slices of chorizo
8 small beef meatballs
1 teaspoon olive oil
10 gr butter
1 tablespoon vegetable bouillon or 1 stock cube
8 toothpicks
1/2 pint of water
Method:
Wash the Brussels sprouts, take out any bruised outer leaves and cut in half lengthways (keep the stem on both cut halves).

Prepare a vegetable stock with 1/2 pint of water and either 1 tablespoon of vegetable bouillon or 1 stock cube. When the stock is simmering, poach the halved Brussels sprouts and the beef meatballs for 3 minutes. After poaching, set the sprouts and meatballs to one side.

Assemble the mini burgers putting a toothpick through one half sprout, then a slice of chorizo, meatball, another slice of chorizo and finish with another half sprout.

Once all the mini burgers are done, pour the olive oil onto a baking tray, place the mini burgers on the tray and finish with the butter divided into small pieces on top of the mini burgers.

Cook in a 200 degree oven for 15 minutes (check after 10 minutes as if the burgers are very small they might be ready in 10-12 minutes). The sprouts should be slightly crispy and the meat cooked through.

### Spaghetti with Celeriac, Mushrooms and Pomegranate
Ingredients:
1/2 pomegranate
1/4 celeriac
1 Portabello mushroom
1 clove garlic
3 tablespoons olive oil
1 teaspoon capers
80 gr wholemeal spaghetti (for 1 person)
1 pinch salt and pepper
Method:
Boil the celeriac for about 15-20 minutes or until fork-tender.

Gently fry some chopped garlic and the capers in 2 tablespoons of olive oil for 2 minutes then set aside. In the same pan, throw in the chopped celeriac and mushrooms.

Cook for 5-10 minutes until the mushrooms have lost all the excess liquid and the celeriac looks slightly caramelised. Leave to cool and in the meantime cook the spaghetti in salted boiling water (10 minutes or less).

Once the celeriac mixture is cooler, blend to a paste. Drain the pasta when ready then heat the garlic and capers you set aside earlier, add the celeriac sauce and the pasta.

To serve, scatter some pomegranate seeds and add a pinch of salt and pepper to taste with a final flourish of olive oil.

## Roasted Pumpkin, Garlic and Pepper soup
Ingredients:
1 orange or yellow pepper
300gr fresh pumpkin
2 whole cloves of garlic with the skin
1 tablespoon olive oil
1/2 teaspoon curry powder
1 pinch Himalayan salt (pink salt)
1 pinch mixed herbs (oregano etc.)
1/2 litre water
Method:
Roast the garlic, sliced and peeled pumpkin and de-seeded and sliced orange pepper on a tray with a drizzle of olive oil in the oven at 200 degrees for about 15 minutes.

Transfer all the roast vegetables to a pan and add 1/2 litre boiling water, the herbs, salt and curry powder. Cook for another 15-20 minutes, blend and serve.

## Rose hip Ice Lollies
Ingredients:
50 grams fresh or dried rose hip (or rose hip tea bags)
1 tablespoon sugar
Method:
Prepare 0.5 litre (about 1 pint) of rose hip tea with 0.5 litre of boiled water and 50 grams of dried rose hips (or fresh ones depending on the season).

Leave to infuse, add the sugar and cool down for 30 minutes then pour into ice lolly moulds. Put in the freezer for at least 4 hours before serving.

## Rose hip Syrup
Ingredients:
1 lt water
1 kg rose hips
500 gr sugar
Method:
Boil 1 lt of water with the sugar on a medium heat for about 5 minutes until all the sugar is dissolved.

Blitz the rose hip in a blender if fresh or rehydrate the dried berries in a bit of hot water for a couple of minutes and then blend.

Add the rose hips to the simmering sugar syrup and cook slowly on a low heat for 15 minutes.

Strain the mixture twice using a muslin cloth and pour into sterilised bottles.

Keep in a cool place and keep in the fridge once opened.

## Moroccan Turkey Kebab Recipe

Ingredients:

300g turkey breast, diced

4 fresh dates

2 plums

1 small onion

1 teaspoon Manuka honey

2 tablespoons soy sauce

150g yellow lentils

150g quinoa

1 tablespoon vegetable bouillon or 4 cups of fresh vegetable stock

Method:

Quarter the plums and the onion, halve the dates.

Get the skewers and alternate pieces of date, turkey, onion, turkey, plum, turkey and date.

In the meantime prepare the marinade for the skewers: in a pan mix the honey and the soy sauce plus a bit of water, reduce until it becomes slightly sticky (about 5 minutes). Set aside.

Rinse the quinoa and lentils in cold water, drain, then add fresh water to the pan with the quinoa and lentils and cook for 20 minutes. Add the vegetable bouillon or stock.

Grill the skewers until cooked (15-20 mins), turn over a few times and cover with the marinade often.

Serve the skewers on top of the lentils and quinoa and enjoy.

## Lettuce Wraps with Lamb

Ingredients:

80gr lamb mince

4 lettuce leaves

2 shallots

1 pinch salt

1 pinch turmeric
1 pinch chilli flakes
1 tbs coconut oil or other oil/butter with high smoke point
Method:
Gently pan fry the shallots, chopped, in a little coconut oil for 3-5 minutes; when golden, add the lamb mince and cook through (about 10 minutes). Add the seasoning and put aside.
Wash and separate the lettuce leaves, then spoon the lamb mixture on each leaf.

**Elderflower Cordial (inspired by Mary Berry)**
Ingredients:
2½ kg sugar
2 unwaxed lemons
20 fresh elderflower heads (no stalks)
85g citric acid (from chemists), optional
Method:
In a large pan, add the sugar and 1.5 litres of water and bring to a simmer on medium heat but avoid boiling the mixture. Stir every so often.
Slice the lemons thinly. Wash the elderflower and discard any flowers that are covered in bugs or don't look healthy. Shake the flowers gently to remove excess water.
Bring the sugar syrup to the boil, turn off the heat and add the elderflowers, lemon peel and slices and the citric acid (when I prepared the cordial I didn't get the citric acid as I was going to consume it straight away but I do suggest to add it for better preserving). Mix with a wooden spoon to combine all ingredients and cover the pan with a lid, letting everything infuse for 24 hours.

The day after, prepare a large pan or a large bowl where you will transfer the cordial, pour the syrup with a ladle into the bowl filtering it first through a muslin (use a colander to avoid making a mess).
The flowers could be added to a smoothie or a cake, if you like.
Pour the cordial into sterilised bottles using a funnel covered with a muslin cloth to ensure the syrup is clear. To sterilise the bottles, either was with very hot water or use the highest temperature in the dishwasher.

You can drink the cordial straight away diluted in still or sparkling water and you can keep it in the fridge for 6 weeks or keep it in the freezer in ice cube trays and add to drinks.

**Vegetables Wrap aka Veggie Fajita**
Ingredients:
1 red onion, sliced
2 cloves garlic
50 gr sprouting broccoli, cut into pieces
50 gr butternut squash, chopped
1 tablespoon olive oil
1/2 teaspoon curry powder (or Cajun/fajita spice mix)
1 spring onion, chopped
1 tortilla wrap
Method:
In a frying pan, gently heat the curry (or Cajun) spice mix with the olive oil over a medium heat for one minute. Add the sprouting broccoli, garlic, red onion and butternut squash and fry for 10 minutes (or until tender) over a high heat.
Add the spring onion and cook for one more minute. Remove all vegetables from the pan and set aside; toast the wrap in the pan for a few seconds, add the vegetables and roll up. Turn the wrap over onto the other side, toast for a few seconds and serve.
For a Tex Mex fajita version serve with guacamole and sour cream.

**Grilled Chicken with fresh Dates and Chicory**
Ingredients:
1 chicken breast
1 head of chicory
10 fresh dates
Soy sauce
Demerara sugar
1 clove garlic
1 small red chilli
Parsley
Olive oil
Method:

Cut the chicory into quarters and the dates in half removing the stones. Place on a baking tray and add 1 tablespoon of water, 1 tablespoon of soy sauce, sprinkle 1/2 teaspoon of Demerara sugar and 1 tablespoon of olive oil.

Put under the grill for about 10 minutes and turn over half way. Check that the sugar caramelises without burning.

In the meantime chop the garlic, chilli and flat leaf parsley (about 5 leaves) and sprinkle over the chicken breast.

Place the prepared chicken over the chicory and dates and cook through turning it over half way (total cooking time 15-20 minutes depending on thickness).

## Chinese Steamed Buns with Lamb

Ingredients:

100 gr braising lamb, cubed

50 gr borlotti beans

5 gr Cajun seasoning

5 gr vegetable bouillon powder

50 gr Kalamata olives

50 gr tomato passata

5 gr Cayenne pepper

7 tablespoons self-raising flour (about 120 gr)

4 tablespoons soya milk or semi-skimmed milk (about 80 gr)

1 pinch of salt

oil for greasing

Method:

For the filling: in a pan on a low heat add the lamb, olives, tomatoes, beans, Cayenne, bouillon and cook for 2 hours until tender.

For the dumplings: mix the self-raising flour with the soya milk and a pinch of salt. Knead until the mixture is not sticky and form 4 balls the size of tennis balls.

Assembly: get 2 fairy cake cases (paper cases) per dumpling, lightly grease them with oil. Get one ball of dough and hollow it in the middle, placing 1 teaspoon of lamb filling in the centre. Fold the rim of the dough around the filling and place into the paper cups.

Cooking: use a steamer or put a steaming basket over a pan of boiling water. Cook for 15 minutes (or 20 minutes if the dough still feels uncooked at the touch).

## Easy Mushroom and Chestnut Soup
Ingredients:
2 chestnut mushrooms, sliced
3 baby potatoes, sliced
3 teaspoons chestnut purée (or 6 whole cooked chestnuts)
1 teaspoon olive oil
2 cloves garlic, chopped
1 tablespoon vegetable bouillon
1 teaspoon mixed herbs (oregano/herbs de Provence)
Method:
Gently fry the garlic in oil for about 3 minutes to infuse the oil. Add the mushrooms and cook for 5 minutes to release some of their water. Add the potatoes and chestnut purée, cook for a further 5 minutes stirring constantly to prevent sticking.
Dissolve the vegetable bouillon in hot water, then add to the vegetables together with the aromatic herbs. Cook for 15 minutes until the potatoes are soft. You can blend the soup for a smoother consistency.

## Asian-Style Coconut Chicken Nuggets with Chilli Dipping Sauce
Ingredients:
1 chicken breast cut into chunks
1 egg yolk
2 tablespoons cornflour
2 tablespoons desiccated coconut
1 pinch of salt and pepper
1 tablespoon olive oil
Dipping sauce:
3 tablespoons apple cider vinegar
1 tablespoon sugar
1/2 teaspoon dried chillies (or 1 fresh chilli)
1 tablespoon soy sauce
Method:
Prepare 3 different bowls and put egg yolk in one, cornflour in one and coconut in the other.
Dip the chicken pieces in cornflour first, egg second and coconut

third.

Place the chicken in an oiled roasting tray and cook in the oven at 180 degrees for 20-30 minutes depending on how big the pieces are.

Meanwhile heat the sugar, chilli, vinegar and soy sauce in a pan on a medium heat for 3-5 minutes ensuring the liquid doesn't evaporate too much. If you prefer a syrupy dipping sauce cook for slightly longer but keep an eye on the pan as it may burn.

Serve the chicken with the dipping sauce with a side of green beans or a salad.

# SOURCES

Chapter 1

Sharples, R. W., Peripatetic Philosophy, 200 BC to AD 200: An Introduction and Collection of Sources in Translation (Cambridge Source Books in Post-Hellenistic Philosophy)

Gardner, Robert M., On Trying To Teach: The Mind in Correspondence

Calories per Hour
http://www.caloriesperhour.com/tutorial_pound.php

Abdominal fat and degenerative health diseases
http://www.health.harvard.edu/fhg/updates/abdominal-obesity-and-your-health.shtml

Walking is no longer the exercise underdog
http://www.healthgreatness.com/healthy-tips/walking-longer-exercise-underdog/

Slow and fast twitch muscles
http://www.bbc.co.uk/science/humanbody/body/factfiles/fastandslowtwitch/soleus.shtml

Hardy, Leah, and Rogers, Susie, Your Hormone Doctor

Waist measurements and diabetes
http://www.bbc.co.uk/news/health-28564566

Posture and state of mind
http://www.elephantjournal.com/2010/05/buddhism-50-of-your-state-of-mind-is-dependent-on-your-posture/

Map My Walk app

My Fitness Pal app

Article: Walking makes workers more resilient to stress
http://www.bbc.co.uk/news/health-29175088

Chapter 2

Why diets don't work, Forbes
http://www.forbes.com/sites/nextavenue/2013/11/19/why-diets-dont-work-and-what-to-do-instead/

What are you Hungry for, Deepak Chopra
The facts about weight loss products & programs, Attorney General
http://www.attorneygeneral.gov/uploadedfiles/consumers/weight_loss.pdf

Empty calories http://www.choosemyplate.gov/preschoolers/daily-food-plans/about-empty-calories.html

National Diabetes Information Clearinghouse (NDIC), A service of the National Institute of Diabetes and Digestive and Kidney Diseases (NIDDK), National Institutes of Health (NIH)
http://diabetes.niddk.nih.gov/dm/pubs/insulinresistance/

I quit sugar http://iquitsugar.com/blog/

Against all grain http://againstallgrain.com/

Comparative study on diets
http://www.nejm.org/doi/full/10.1056/NEJMoa0804748

Criticism of paleo diet http://www.smh.com.au/lifestyle/diet-and-fitness/nutritionists-warn-of-dangers-in-paleo-dieting-20140805-100iup.html

The truth about crabs

http://www.nhs.uk/livewell/loseweight/pages/the-truth-about-carbs.aspx

Atkins, Robert C., Dr Atkins New Diet Revolution: The No-hunger, Luxurious Weight Loss Plan That Really Works!

Cordain, Loren, The Paleo Diet: Lose Weight and Get Healthy by Eating the Foods You Were Designed to Eat

D'Adamo, Peter, Eat Right 4 Your Type

Gallop, Rick, The Gi Diet: The Glycemic Index; The Easy, Healthy Way to Permanent Weight Loss

Mosley, Dr Michael, The Fast Diet: The Secret of Intermittent Fasting – Lose Weight, Stay Healthy, Live Longer

Norris, Jack, Vegan for Life: Everything You Need to Know to Be Healthy and Fit on a Plant-Based Diet

Sears, Barry, Enter The Zone - A Dietary Road Map to Lose Weight Permanently

Panagos, Angelique, Article: Eating disorders, hypothyroidism, PCOS, fertility, conception & miscarriage

Angelique Panagos website:  http://angeliquepanagos.com/

Chapter 3

Huffington, Arianna, Thrive: The Third Metric to Redefining Success and Creating a Happier Life

Balding, Clare, Walking Home: My Family and Other Rambles

Forage London website http://www.foragelondon.co.uk/

Health benefits of malic acid

http://www.thehealthierlife.co.uk/natural-health-articles/chronic-fatigue-syndrome/malic-acid-chronic-fatigue-syndrome-00974/

London parks, 75 km walk from Croydon to Barnet
http://ravenellison.com/2014/06/08/children-are-like-an-endangered-species-in-many-of-londons-woods/

London is 47% green space
http://www.independent.co.uk/environment/47-per-cent-of-london-is-green-space-is-it-time-for-our-capital-to-become-a-national-park-9756470.html

Rensten, John, Article: Elongated seasons: Springtime in November http://www.foragelondon.co.uk/spring-time-in-november/

Rensten, John, Article: Wild food is super food
http://www.foragelondon.co.uk/wild-food-is-super-food/

Rensten, John, Article: Easily identify 4 late season wild mushrooms http://www.foragelondon.co.uk/learn-to-safely-id-these-4-late-season-wild-mushrooms/

Fletcher, Neil, The Easy Wild Food Guide

Mabey, Richard, Food for free

Phillips, Roger, Wild Food: A Complete Guide for Foragers

Phillips, Roger, Mushrooms

Wright, John, Hedgerow (River Cottage Handbook, No.7)

Wright, John, Mushrooms: River Cottage Handbook No.1

Bassanese, Paola, Article: Plant power and properties
http://www.energyanaturalfacelift.com/2014/06/herbalist-walk-plant-power-and-properties/

London Walks http://www.walks.com/London_Walks_Home

Highgate Woods guided walks https://www.cityoflondon.gov.uk

Oakdown Holiday Park http://www.oakdown.co.uk/index.html winner of the David Bellamy Gold Environmental Awards

Berry Quarry caves in East Devon http://beerquarrycaves.co.uk/

Sophrology resources: http://www.be-sophro.co.uk and http://www.sophroacademy.co.uk/

Parrot, Florence, Instant Serenity for Life and Work

Stiegler, Edouard-G., Régénération par la marche afghane

Tolle, Eckhart, The Power of Now: A Guide to Spiritual Enlightenment
Weisman, Arinna, and Smith, Jane, The Beginner's Guide to Insight Meditation

Zanin, Daniel, website: http://www.marche-consciente.com/


Wikipedia: Walking Meditation How To
http://www.wikihow.com/Do-Walking-Meditation

Article: Health benefits of walking
http://www.heart.org/HEARTORG/GettingHealthy/PhysicalActivity/StartWalking/Physical-activity-improves-quality-of-life_UCM_307977_Article.jsp

Article: Walking beneficial for Alzheimer's
http://www.webmd.com/alzheimers/news/20101128/walking-may-cut-alzheimers-risk

I Quit Sugar: Your Complete 8-Week Detox Program and Cookbook, Sarah Wilson

Health benefits of walking WHO report
http://www.euro.who.int/en/health-topics/environment-and-health/Transport-and-health/activities/guidance-and-tools/health-economic-assessment-tool-heat-for-cycling-and-walking

Walking a mile a day can cut risk of dying from cancer by 40%
http://www.theguardian.com/society/2014/aug/29/walking-mile-day-cut-risk-dying-breast-prostate-cancer-40pc?CMP=twt_gu

Rodgers, Nile: Walking on Planet C blog
http://www.nilerodgers.com/blogs

Future Green Studio http://futuregreenstudio.com/research/

Society of Young Publishers http://thesyp.org.uk/

Article:  Walk this way for fitness

Dominique Antiglio website: http://www.be-sophro.co.uk/

Joanna Hall website: http://www.joannahall.com/

Tracey Cox website:  http://www.traceycox.com/about/

## ABOUT THE AUTHOR

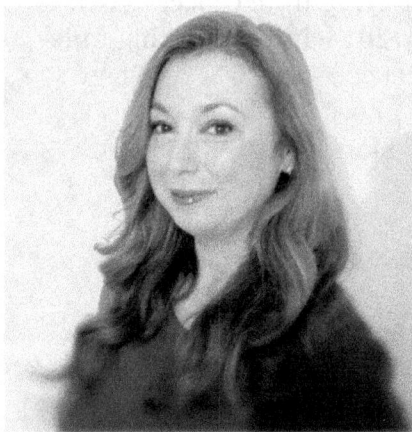 Paola Bassanese, MA IR/ES, ITEC Dip., is the owner and director of Energya Ltd, a company specialising in stress management solutions.

After a 15 year career in the corporate world and an inspirational trip to Peru, she founded Energya Ltd to provide high quality wellness services to a loyal customer base.

As an author, Paola has written for the international consultancy Ovum and for the Economist, she was quoted in the Financial Times and her story was published in Spirit and Destiny. She had articles published in the Huffington Post in the UK Lifestyle section and MassageSchool.org in the United States.

You may also like to read The Foraging Home Cook, a collection of recipes using foraged ingredients.

You can connect with Paola Bassanese at www.energya.co.uk, on Twitter at @paolaenergya, on LinkedIn and on Google +.